The Definitive Guide to Raising Resilient Children

Empower Your Kids to Master Their Emotions, Solve Problems, Overcome Adversity, and Build Unshakable Confidence

Lee Alexander

© Copyright Lee Alexander 2025 - All rights reserved.

The content within this book may not be reproduced, duplicated or transmitted without direct written permission from the author or the publisher.

Under no circumstances will any blame or legal responsibility be held against the publisher, or author, for any damages, reparation, or monetary loss due to the information contained within this book. Either directly or indirectly. You are responsible for your own choices, actions, and results.

Legal Notice:

This book is copyright-protected. This book is only for personal use. You cannot amend, distribute, sell, use, quote, or paraphrase any part of this book's content without the author's or publisher's consent.

Disclaimer Notice:

Please note the information contained within this document is for educational and entertainment purposes only. All effort has been expended to present accurate, up-to-date, reliable, and complete information. No warranties of any kind are declared or implied. Readers acknowledge that the author is not engaging in rendering legal, financial, medical, or professional advice. The content within this book has been derived from various sources. Please consult a licensed professional before attempting any techniques outlined in this book.

By reading this document, the reader agrees that under no circumstances is the author responsible for any losses, direct or indirect, which are incurred as a result of the use of the information contained within this document, including, but not limited to, — errors, omissions, or inaccuracies.

Contents

Introduction	VII
1. Your Approach Matters	1
2. Attachment and Connection	13
3. Emotions and Empathy	25
4. Growth Mindset	41
5. Thinking, Solving and Deciding	51
Make a Difference With Your Review	61
6. Autonomy and Independence	63
7. Adaptability and Ingenuity	71
8. Conflict	81
9. Hardship	91
10. Parental Resilience	105
Keeping the Journey Going	117
Conclusion	119
References	121
Also by Lee Alexander	133

Introduction

Nine-year-old Sophie lay on her bed, covered in a mound of blankets, proclaiming she would not leave her room for the rest of her life. The piano recital had been a disaster. Halfway through her piece, she had forgotten the notes and stumbled through the rest. Her fingers hit all the wrong keys while the audience sat in polite, awkward silence. Now, in the safety of her room, her emotions overflowed. "I'm terrible! I'll never play again!" she sobs, burying her face in her hands. You kneel beside her, trying to comfort her, but Sophie can't hear anything over the roar of her self-criticism. The weight of failure pressed heavily on her tiny shoulders, and at that moment, it felt like she would never recover.

Situations like Sophie's may resonate with you. As their parent, you want to step in—to shield them from pain, protect them from failure, and fight their battles for them. Yet deep down, you know that life's challenges will not always be as simple or short-lived as a poor piano performance. Today's world is demanding and complex, filled with pressures that stretch far beyond the recital stage.

Children face immense pressures that were hardly imaginable 30 years ago. They face consumerism, comparison culture, social media traps, drugs, and more, all mixed up in a fast-paced, uncertain world. Mental health concerns have risen sharply, especially in the pandemic's aftermath. The career landscape is highly competitive, and the cost of living is high. There are more temptations to stray off the noble path than ever before.

These realities make it more important than ever to prepare children to survive into and through adulthood. But don't you want them to do more than just survive? You want them to *thrive*. You want them to be happy. You want them to support themselves and not live with you forever. You want them to reach their highest potential. This can only happen if you equip them with resilience now.

Research agrees that resilient children do better in the long run. They outperform their peers academically, have better interpersonal relationships, and are more equipped to handle life's hurdles. So, you know these qualities are crucial for lifelong success, but you might be wondering, what exactly is resilience? How can you tell if children have it or they don't? What special training or courses are required to instill it? How much time and money is this going to take? And most importantly, how do you nurture it in your children if you don't feel very resilient yourself?

Human resilience is the capacity to **adapt** effectively through adversity, trauma, or significant stress. It involves mental, emotional, and behavioral **flexibility** and **adjusting** to external and internal demands. Key components include **emotional regulation, problem-solving skills, social support**, and **optimism.**

If you've ever worried that your child just isn't resilient or struggles more than others, you're not alone—but there is good news. Resilience is not a "have" or "have not" trait that some people are born with and some are not. You can cultivate resilience through experiences, learning, and intentional practices. This means that every child can develop and increase these skills, no matter who they are, where they come from, or what start they got in life.

The required parental skills are love, presence, and willingness to try. It costs nothing, and you'll be surprised how little time it actually takes. This book offers the strategies you need to build these traits today, resulting in a dramatically different household in no time.

Being a "good" parent is not about shielding children from stress or ensuring they never experience hardship. Instead, it means arming them with the ability to face their fears, learn from failure, and continue pushing forward. This distinction is critical because your role as a parent is not to eliminate every obstacle in your children's path. Your role is to prepare them to face these obstacles bravely and, if they fail, to get back up stronger than before.

You won't always be there to protect them and fight their battles. This much is certain. But you can empower them today to stand strong, adapt, and persevere independently. Then they will be ready to tackle life on their own when you are gone.

Inside this book, you will discover practical, evidenced-based strategies to help develop strength, grit, and tenacity in your children. You'll learn how to create an environment that supports emotional fortitude, fosters problem-solving skills, and encourages a growth mindset. You'll also discover how to nurture resilience in yourself, because your actions play a central role in shaping your children.

Building confident and capable children is not a quick, one-and-done approach. It is a gradual, ongoing process that requires patience and intentionality. But the rewards are profound.

Resilient children grow into strong adults who can navigate life's complexities with courage, determination, and hope. You have everything you need right now to make this happen. Change is within reach. With this book as a guide, you can empower the next generation to rise above their challenges, embrace change, and build a healthy foundation that will serve them for a lifetime. Let's get started.

Chapter One

Your Approach Matters

Children are not one-size-fits-all. Each one comes into the world with a unique blend of tendencies, temperaments, and ways of interacting with their environment. Even siblings raised in the same household can exhibit vastly different personalities, preferences, and needs. The influence of genetics, environmental factors, and individual experiences is far from completely understood. Building resilience in children begins with understanding and embracing these differences.

Tailoring your parenting approach to each child is crucial for meeting their distinct needs, nurturing their strengths, and encouraging their growth. This chapter delves into practical tools for adapting your parenting style, refining communication strategies, and offering personalized support. It's about discovering what resonates with your children and empowering them to blossom as their most authentic selves.

Parental Attitudes

Your child stands at the playground's edge, hesitating, yet eager to climb the jungle gym for the first time. You watch, and your heart is a mix of hope and worry. They look back at you with excitement, fear, and doubt in their eyes. They're waiting for you to say something. What should you say?

In this pivotal moment, your words—whether an assertive "You can do it!" or a cautious "Be careful!"—set the tone for how your children approach this and all future challenges. These seemingly small choices in language and attitude play a significant role in shaping character and self-efficacy.

As a parent, your outlook becomes the lens through which your children view the world. Whether or not you realize it, your attitudes and reactions profoundly influence them. Children are sponges, always watching, learning, and internalizing.

Which mindset do you want to convey? What impression do you want your words to leave on them? How do you want your children to view the world and their place in it?

Your words, tone, inflection, and body language shape how your children see themselves and their environment. When parents frequently express negativity or hopelessness, children may view hardship and failure as insurmountable. This promotes a belief that they are not in control of their lives; that their efforts toward success are futile, subject to the chaotic play of the universe.

With this paradigm internalized, children may interpret stumbling blocks as evidence of their inadequacy instead of opportunities for improvement. Dismissive or critical language, such as "You'll never get it right!" or "Why can't you be more like others?" can further erode children's self-worth and confidence.

This type of language diminishes their motivation and instills a fear of mistakes, stifling creativity, and discouraging them from taking risks.

Conversely, intentionally choosing positive and supportive words can shift the narrative entirely. Children raised in an environment where good faith and optimism are consistently shown are more likely to develop these qualities. Affirming language, such as "I believe in you!" or "You handled that well!" can empower children, lifting their spirit and encouraging a positive attitude. Setbacks are seen as temporary and manageable.

This environment reinforces children's self-esteem, empowering them to face dilemmas with optimism and perseverance. It teaches them that they are the ones in control of their destiny.

Reflection Exercise

Do I approach life with an open heart or a guarded stance?

Do I generally expect good outcomes or focus on what might go wrong?

Do I worry alot, or trust that things will work out?

Do I surround myself with people who uplift and support me?

Do I actively engage with negativity?

How do I measure success?

What kind of person do I want to be remembered as?

Parental Behavior

The behaviors that children see in their parents often become a template for their own conduct. When you model honorable behavior, it teaches your children lessons that words alone cannot convey. Telling your children one thing while behaving in a contradictory way doesn't work. Actions speak louder than words. Your children will always mimic your behavior rather than your words.

Imagine a parent caught in heavy traffic, the frustration palpable. Instead of honking and grumbling, they take a deep breath, choose an uplifting song, and explain to their children why staying calm is important. This simple act becomes a significant lesson in emotional regulation. It shows children how to manage stress and cope with troubles, teaching them that reactions are choices, not reflexes.

The key is consistency. Occasional respect and kindness are valuable, but the long-term impact comes from a sustained effort to model patience, compassion, and tranquility. Children thrive when they see these qualities repeatedly demonstrated in everyday life, from how you manage minor inconveniences to how you celebrate achievements.

This consistency emphasizes that these attitudes are not just situational, but deeply embedded into the core of your psyche and family culture. Children learn by example. Your calm and respectful behavior will teach them to build healthier relationships. This will help them better handle conflicts and challenges in their own lives.

Reflection Exercise

How do I show kindness and appreciation to the people in my life?

Do I let frustration overshadow the bigger picture of what's going well?

How do I typically react when I'm stressed or frustrated?

Do I control my emotions before responding to challenging situations?

What tone of voice and body language do I use when I'm upset?

Am I modeling the respect I expect my children to show to others?

How often do I apologize when I make a mistake?

Are there situations where I wish I had responded differently?

Parenting Styles

Being aware of your parenting style can profoundly affect your family dynamics and children's development. The primary parenting styles[1] are Authoritative, Permissive, Uninvolved and Authoritarian (Amato & Fowler, 2002; Laff & Ruiz, 2019). Each style reflects different approaches to discipline, communication, and warmth. Understanding these styles can help you assess and improve your parenting approach to benefit your children's development.

Authoritarian (strict approach) is characterized by high expectations and low responsiveness. The system enforces strict rules with little explanation or flexibility. Communication is primarily one-sided, with an emphasis on obedience rather than understanding. Discipline is often punitive rather than instructive. The drawback of this approach is that children may become obedient but struggle with self-esteem and decision-making. They may develop anxiety, resentment, or defiance over time.

Permissive (lenient) parenting involves a high level of responsiveness but low expectations. These parents often indulge their children, providing few rules or boundaries. They are nurturing and communicative, but may struggle with enforcing discipline. They avoid confrontation and often prioritize their children's happiness over setting limits. The consequence of this approach is that children may struggle with self-discipline and respect for authority. They might exhibit behavioral problems and find it hard to cope with stress.

Uninvolved (neglectful) parenting is characterized by low warmth and low control. Parents in this category provide minimal guidance, emotional support, or supervision. Unlike other parenting styles, neglectful parents are largely disengaged from their child's life, often due to stress, personal struggles, or a lack of understanding about the importance of active parenting. Neglectful parenting can have serious consequences for a child's emotional, social, and cognitive development including low self-esteem, behavioral issues and difficulty forming relationships.

Authoritative parenting (balanced approach) comprises high responsiveness and high expectations. Parents set clear rules and guidelines, explaining the reasons behind them. These parents encourage open communication and support their children's needs and emotions. Discipline is consistent and based on educating rather than punishing. Children are self-reliant, socially competent, and emotionally

---

1. As first described by Baumrind and later expanded upon by Maccoby and Martin.

secure. They perform well academically and have strong problem-solving skills.

A balanced parenting style can create a loving environment that encourages children to flourish. They learn to respect boundaries while feeling supported and understood. This balance helps to equip them with the skills to face hurdles with courage and adaptability. The will grow to respect themselves more as well as those in positions of authority.

Determining Your Parenting Style

Authoritative

Do I enforce rules strictly without explaining their purpose?

Is obedience more important than understanding my children's feelings?

Do I often use punishment rather than teaching as a disciplinary method?

Permissive

Do I often give in to my children's demands to avoid conflict?

Am I inconsistent with setting and enforcing rules or boundaries?

Do I prioritize my children's happiness over teaching responsibility?

Uninvolved

Do I use screens as a substitute for direct interaction with my children?

Do I leave them alone for extended periods without checking in?

Do I prioritize work, social life, or personal issues over spending time with them?

Authoritative

Do I provide clear expectations and explain the reasons behind them?

Am I responsive to their emotions while maintaining boundaries?

Do I encourage my children to express their thoughts and opinions?

Parenting is one of the hardest jobs in the world, and reflecting on our parenting style can sometimes bring up feelings of guilt or regret. But the goal of examining this topic is **not** to shame or criticize—it's to bring awareness and growth. Many parents struggle with exhaustion, stress, or life circumstances that make it challenging to be as engaged as they'd like. If you recognize patterns of neglectful parenting in your own life, it doesn't mean you're a bad parent—it simply means there's an opportunity to make positive changes. Every parent has moments where they fall short, but what matters most is the willingness to reflect, learn, and take small steps toward greater connection and support for your children. Parenting is a journey, and no one gets it perfect all the time.

Introverts/Extroverts

Personality traits are what make each person unique. Traits include elements such as thoughts, feelings, behaviors, and patterns of interacting with the world. Introversion and extroversion are key components of personality.

The tendency toward either introversion or extroversion explains how individuals gain energy, approach relationships, and engage with their surroundings. Many individuals fall between these extremes, exhibiting traits from both ends of the spectrum. By understanding whether your children tend toward introversion or extroversion, you can align your expectations and interactions with their personality. This will increase their trust and cooperation and strengthen your bond.

Introversion is characterized by a preference for internal thoughts and feelings over social interactions. Introverts feel energized and rejuvenated after spending time alone. They are highly sensitive to external stimulation, such as large social gatherings, which can feel overwhelming. This leads them to seek environments with minimal distractions. They choose quiet, reflective activities like reading or writing. They find these activities more fulfilling than the hustle and noise of social events.

Introverts are thoughtful and deliberate, often preferring meaningful conversations over small talk. Rather than maintaining a large circle of acquaintances, introverts usually invest in a few close relationships with people who are authentic, reliable, and emotionally present. They avoid conflict, preferring harmonious environments. They retreat from confrontational situations when they arise.

Extroverts draw energy from social interactions and external stimuli, often exhibiting outgoing and enthusiastic behaviors. They thrive in group settings, finding fulfillment in engaging with others and taking part in communal activities. These settings allow them to develop interpersonal skills and learn to navigate social dynamics. Extroverts benefit from environments where they can voice their thoughts and influence the group. They may experience restlessness or depletion during prolonged periods of solitude.

Key characteristics of extroverts include sociability, assertiveness, and talkativeness. They are often comfortable starting conversations and enjoy being at the center of attention. Their commanding nature enables them to express opinions confidently and take leadership roles in group scenarios. Extroverts are action-oriented, preferring to engage actively with their environment rather than spending extensive time in reflection. They are adaptable and can easily navigate new or changing situations, often seeking excitement and variety in their experiences.

Determining Introversion/Extroversion in Your Children

How do my children react to new situations?

How do they handle meeting new people?

Do they prefer a set routine? Or embrace spontaneity?

Do they share their thoughts and feelings openly or keep them private?

Do they talk through their thoughts or process internally before sharing?

How do they react to periods of solitude?

After a social gathering, are they energized or drained?

Learning Styles

There are many ways that individuals learn. Though it is not impossible to learn through other methods, using a person's preferred method can significantly enhance the educational experience. Recognizing your children's primary learning style allows you to create more effective and engaging ways to help them with homework, explore novel topics, and develop new skills. It makes learning more enjoyable, helps them grasp concepts more efficiently, and builds certainty in their abilities.

The VARK Model, as first described by Fleming and Mills, identifies four primary learning styles: visual, auditory, reading, and kinesthetic (VARK Learn Limited, 2024).

Visual learners prefer to process information through images, diagrams, charts, algorithms, and other pictographic aids. They benefit from seeing concepts mapped out and often use visualization techniques to remember information.

Auditory learners absorb information best through listening. They learn effectively through lectures, discussions, and audio materials and may prefer reading aloud or using mnemonic devices involving sound.

Reading/writing learners favor interacting with text. They excel through reading and writing activities, such as note-taking, reading articles, and engaging with written explanations.

Kinesthetic learners prefer a hands-on approach, lived experience, and opportunities to practice skills. They benefit from activities that involve movement, experiments, and real-life examples.

Beyond the VARK model, Gardner has proposed additional learning styles (Multiple Intelligences Oasis, n.d.):

Logical learners thrive on facts, reasoning, and frameworks. They like analyzing the structure of arguments, looking for patterns, and forming conclusions based on the validity and soundness of the evidence. People most commonly apply these principles in philosophy, mathematics, and computer science.

Social learners prefer to engage with others and take part in collaborative activities. These individuals learn best when sharing ideas, discussing concepts, and working with peers. They may excel in situations where they can teach or explain concepts to others, reinforcing their understanding and knowledge.

Solitary learners favor self-study and introspection and learn best when working alone.

Determining Your Children's Learning Style

Visual

Do my children enjoy looking at pictures, diagrams, or videos to understand a concept?

Do they use color coding or drawing to organize their thoughts?

Auditory

Do they prefer listening to explanations rather than reading instructions?

Do they remember songs, rhymes, or verbal cues more quickly than visual information?

Reading

Do they enjoy reading books or writing notes, lists, or stories?

Do they retain information better after writing it down or reading it?

Kinesthetic

Do they prefer hands-on activities like crafting or experimenting?

Are they more engaged when physically moving or manipulating objects?

Social/Solitary

Do they prefer working independently or in small groups?

Love Languages

This concept describes five primary ways individuals give and receive love (Chapman & Campbell, 2016). Understanding your children's love language can significantly enhance your bond. Children feel genuinely valued and understood when you use their primary love language. By tailoring your approach to meet their unique emotional needs, you can cultivate a deeper connection and strengthen trust.

Children who value **Words of Affirmation** feel loved when they hear positive, encouraging, and validating words. They need compliments, praise, or expressions of love such as "I'm proud of you!" or "I love you." These children flourish on verbal reinforcement and may feel unappreciated or unloved without it. Positive affirmations build their confidence and emotional resolve. Examples of statements these children would find valuable include, "You're making great progress—keep it up!" and "You can do it!!—I believe in you!"

For children who value **Quality Time**, your undivided attention is the ultimate expression of affection. They treasure shared experiences and one-on-one sessions where they feel prioritized. Neglecting quality time can lead these children to feel disconnected or ignored. Togetherness deepens your bond and gives them a sense of security. Consider scheduling regular parent-child dates where you focus entirely on them, such as going for a walk, playing a game, or cooking together.

Children who value **Acts of Service** feel loved when you do things for them, like helping with homework, preparing their favorite meal, or assisting with a challenging task. These children interpret helpful and thoughtful deeds as expressions of care. Consistent acts of service show them they're supported and valued. Help them prepare for a big school presentation by practicing with them or organizing their materials.

For children who value **Physical Touch**, hugs, cuddles, high-fives, or a reassuring pat on the back make them feel loved and secure. These children value physical closeness. Without it, they may feel disconnected or unloved. Give them a warm hug after a long day, let them sit on your lap during a movie or hold their hand while crossing the street.

Children who value **Receiving Gifts** feel loved through thoughtful, tangible symbols of affection. The meaning behind the gift matters more than its monetary value. Gifts are a visual reminder of love and care. Neglecting this love language might lead them to feel overlooked or insignificant. Surprise them with a small, thoughtful gift like a handwritten note, a favorite snack, or an item they've been wishing for.

Children who feel consistently and unconditionally loved are more likely to develop strong self-esteem, emotional fortitude, and healthy, secure relationships. Even the most well-intentioned expressions of love can sometimes miss the mark if they don't align with how a child perceives love. Utilizing their preferred language ensures your children recognize and internalize your love, the precursor to their emotional and social growth. It will also minimize misunderstandings and build a base of trust.

Determining Your Children's Love Language

Quality Time

Do my children frequently ask to spend time with me?

Do they light up when I give them my undivided attention, even briefly?

How do they react when I am busy or distracted?

What activities do they ask to do with me the most?

Words of Affirmation

Do they frequently seek verbal praise or reassurance from me?

How do they respond to compliments or encouragement?

Do they remember kind words or seem hurt by criticism?

Acts of Service

Do my children ask for help with tasks, even if they could do them alone?

How do they respond when I go out of my way to assist them?

Do they show appreciation when I do something nice for them?

When upset, do they seem comforted by actions rather than words?

Physical Touch

Do my children often initiate physical contact with me?

Do they seek comfort through physical touch when upset or scared?

How do they react to playful physical interactions, like tickling or wrestling?

Do they express disappointment if I don't hug or kiss them goodbye?

Receiving Gifts

Do my children light up when receiving a thoughtful gift?

Do they cherish the items I give them and treat them with great care?

How do they react when they are surprised with an unexpected present?

Do they frequently make or give gifts to others to express love?

Additional Observations

What do they complain about most often? For example, "You never spend time with me" might suggest Quality Time is their preferred language.

How do they naturally express love to others? People often show love in the way they prefer to receive it.

How do they react when they feel unloved? A child who craves Physical Touch may seem withdrawn if they don't get enough cuddles, while a child whose love language is Words of Affirmation may become sensitive to harsh comments.

What activities make them happiest? Pay attention to how they behave during one-on-one time, at family gatherings, or when they receive a gift or help.

Practical Test

Experiment with each love language intentionally and observe their reactions. For example:

- Spend extra time with them one day (Quality Time).
- Give them a small surprise gift (Receiving Gifts).
- Write a heartfelt note (Words of Affirmation).
- Help with a chore (Acts of Service).
- Give extra hugs or pats on the back (Physical Touch).

Summary

Understanding the nuances of your children's personalities and specific needs and preferences is paramount to developing resilience.

Each child's unique blend of traits and experiences requires a tailored approach.

Addressing these differences with sensitivity and support fosters a balanced sense of self, equipping children to face life's problems courageously.

Chapter Two

Attachment and Connection

As a parent, you are far more than a source of comfort to your children. You are their anchor in the ever-changing sea of their self-perception and developing emotions. Your presence provides stability and reassurance during uncertainty, frustration, or fear. The bond you share with your children forms the foundation upon which they build their emotional well-being and capacity for healthy relationships both now and in the future. You are their compass in navigating the complex and often overwhelming experiences of growing up.

Reflection Exercise

Do my children seek comfort from me when upset, hurt, or scared?

Do they willingly share their thoughts, feelings, or experiences with me?

How do they behave when I leave for an extended period?

How do they react when I return after being apart?

Do they show confidence in exploring new situations?

Do I actively listen when they speak, or am I often distracted?

When was the last time I had a meaningful conversation with them?

How do I respond when my children share something important?

Attachment

Early relationships with caregivers have a profound effect on children's sense of security. For infants, the attachment experiences they have with one or two primary caregivers from birth onward create an "internal working model." It is a mental framework for understanding relationships and navigating the world. This model helps children predict and interpret social interactions and guides their behavior in future relationships (Ainsworth, 1978; Bowlby, 1988).

The primary caregiver(s) provide a secure base, enabling children to explore the world fearlessly. This sense of security makes curiosity and experimentation possible. Children feel safe enough to engage with their environment, learn, and connect with others. They know they can return to this secure base for comfort and reassurance should fear, difficulty, hurt, or pain occur.

Secure attachment means caregivers consistently offer children love, affection, and reassurance whenever they require it.

Children with secure attachments often exhibit better emotional regulation and higher self-esteem. These early attachment experiences also significantly impact how they form relationships in adulthood. Securely attached children are more likely to develop healthy, fulfilling relationships as adults, whereas those with insecure attachments may face intimacy, trust, and communication issues.

Parenting plays a pivotal role in the development of attachment. Responsive, sensitive, and emotionally available caregiving help develop a secure attachment. Conversely, parenting that is inconsistent, neglectful, or emotionally unavailable may lead to insecure attachment.

Factors such as parental mental health, emotional availability, and the ability to provide consistent care are crucial in shaping the children's attachment style. For this reason and many others, your health and well-being must be at the forefront so you can care for your children effectively (see Chapter 10).

Increasing Attachment

It's never too early or too late to increase your bond with your children. During **preschool (age 2 to 5)**, children flourish with shared play, consistent routines, and physical affection. Engaging in imaginative play, such as pretend tea parties or dress-up, and games like hide-and-seek helps them know they are worthy enough for you to spend time with.

Establishing rituals, such as reading a favorite bedtime story or singing a lullaby, creates a comforting sense of routine. It can be a special moment of togetherness they can look forward to each day. Physical affection, including hugs, cuddles, and high-fives, are essential for showing love and support, as are simple gestures like eye contact and smiling when they speak. Celebrating their small achievements, such as dressing and combing their hair, boosts their self-esteem.

School-age (age 5 to 10) children are developing independence but still rely on emotional support and shared experiences. Scheduling one-on-one time dedicated to their interests reinforces their sense of importance within the family. Offer guidance with homework or school projects without taking over. This allows them to feel supported while promoting their independent efforts.

Encouraging authentic communication by asking about their day or friendships and actively listening strengthens trust and understanding. Taking part in family activities, such as nature walks, board games, or family movie nights helps maintain a sense of togetherness. Supporting their hobbies by attending sports games, recitals, or other extracurricular events shows your commitment to their passions and builds lasting connections.

As **tweens (age 10 to 12)** seek greater independence, maintaining a strong bond requires a balance of support, understanding, and closeness. Showing genuine interest in their hobbies and asking them to teach you about their interests contributes to mutual respect. Engaging in deeper conversations about their goals, challenges, or current events and creating a judgment-free space for sharing helps build trust and emotional intimacy.

Spending time together on activities like cooking, building, or gardening allows collaboration and connection. Planning outings they enjoy, such as visits to a theme park or museum, create cherished memories. Encouraging their independence by enabling them to make decisions, such as organizing their schedules, validates their developing autonomy.

Stability and Consistency

Children's security and well-being depend on stability and consistency. Stability means providing a predictable, safe, and nurturing environment where children feel supported and convinced of their caregivers' reliability. A stable home environment, free from frequent relocations or significant disruptions, gives them a comforting sense of permanence.

It's equally important to shield children from adult concerns, such as financial or housing issues, as they often internalize these problems and may blame themselves. Maintaining consistency and protecting children from unnecessary stress creates a solid base where they can thrive emotionally and developmentally.

Positive and steady relationships between caregivers and extended family members are fundamental to children's emotional well-being. Even if personal differences exist, maintaining a respectful and cooperative relationship with your children's inner circle is in their best interests. Minimizing their exposure to conflict, arguments, or uncertainty helps create a peaceful and harmonious environment, reducing needless stress and maintaining security and stability.

Consistency in routines, behavior, and emotional responses is key to achieving stability. Regular schedules, such as having set mealtimes, bedtimes, and morning routines, help children know what to expect, providing comfort and predictability. Consistent emotional responses build trust and emotional safety.

Similarly, setting clear expectations, such as limiting screen time or ensuring homework completion before play, helps children understand boundaries and develop self-discipline. You build a healthy infrastructure by consistently responding to their needs and maintaining predictable routines. From this groundwork, children can engage with and be successful in the world outside their nuclear family.

Trust

Trust is the ground upon which all healthy family relationships are built, serving as the bedrock for emotional well-being and security. Children who can count on their parents feel safe, valued, and understood. It provides them a sense of security that allows them to spread their wings. This advances open communication, encouraging children to express their thoughts, feelings, and concerns without fear of judgment or criticism.

In such a supportive environment, children are more willing to take risks and learn from their mistakes, knowing they have a reliable safety net. This alliance strengthens the parent-child bond, sustaining respect and the understanding essential for developing confidence and adaptability as children traverse their world.

Building trust within a family requires consistent effort, honesty, and respect. Reliable actions, like keeping promises and commitments—no matter how small—cultivate trust within families. Whether attending a school event, spending quality time together, or enforcing fair boundaries and consequences, each act reinforces your dependability and accountability. Following through on your word sends a clear message to your children that they can rely on you. Over time, these consistent efforts strengthen family connections and teach children the importance of integrity and fidelity in their relationships.

Trust-building is a gradual process that requires authenticity, active listening, and mutual respect. Keep your promise to pick up your child at the appointed time. If circumstances change, communicate promptly and honestly. Truthfulness, even during difficult situations, models the importance of honesty in relationships. Admitting your mistakes—such as saying, "I'm sorry I overreacted earlier; I should have handled that better."—demonstrates accountability and fosters mutual respect.

As children grow, respecting their boundaries becomes necessary for maintaining trust. Allowing them privacy and autonomy within reasonable limits shows you value their independence and have faith in their judgment. Simple actions, such as knocking before entering their room or refraining from unwarranted prying into their personal lives, demonstrate your respect. This respect encourages them to reciprocate trust, strengthening your relationship and creating an environment where both parties can flourish.

Communication

Every strong and close-knit family has one thing in common: the ability to communicate effectively. When families communicate well, they build bonds that promote mutual respect and understanding. These connections strengthen cooperation. Children can express themselves freely without fear of judgment and feel heard and validated. Creating this communication-rich environment is fundamental in nurturing resilience, as it encourages open dialogue and emotional expression.

Active Listening

What does it mean to actively listen? It requires the listener to give their full attention to the speaker without interruptions or distractions. The listener is trying to understand and remember what the speaker is saying. It means showing genuine interest in their thoughts, feelings, and experiences. It means validating their emotions. This practice reduces misunderstandings, creating a supportive environment for children to share freely.

When you model active listening, children learn to express themselves without fear. Here are some ways you can enhance your active listening skills:

- Give them your undivided attention: Pause what you're doing (e.g., put your phone away and turn off the TV).

- Make eye contact with your children and focus solely on them.

- Show empathy: Acknowledge and validate their emotions by saying things like, "I can see that made you upset," or "It sounds like you're excited about this!"

- Repeat back or summarize what they say to show you understand. Example: "You're upset because your friend didn't share the toy. Is that right?"

- Avoid interrupting: Let your children finish their thoughts before responding.

- Resist the urge to jump in with advice or solutions immediately.

- Respond nonverbally: Use nods, smiles, or a supportive touch to show your listening and engagement.

- Be patient: Allow them time to find the right words, especially if they struggle to express themselves.

- Stay curious: Ask follow-up questions to dig deeper into their feelings or thoughts instead of assuming you know what they are trying to convey.

- Create dedicated "listening time." Set aside a few minutes each day for one-on-one conversations, like during bedtime or a meal, to talk without distractions.

Validation

Affirming your children's feelings as legitimate and understandable is imperative to effective communication. When you validate their experiences, you acknowledge and accept their emotions and thoughts as real and significant, even if you disagree. Validation tells your children that all feelings, even difficult ones, are natural and manageable. This creates a safe emotional environment. They will feel comfortable expressing themselves to you without fear of judgment or dismissal.

Validation doesn't mean agreeing with everything your children say or feel. It's about acknowledging their perspective. Once children feel heard, they are more likely to collaborate to find solutions. Phrases like "I can see why you feel that way" or "That must be hard for you" demonstrate empathy and understanding and can be incredibly de-escalating in a tense situation.

Consider the following example. Your child is frustrated after struggling with a math problem and says, "I'm terrible at math! I'll never get this right!" A validating response from you might be, "I can tell you're feeling frustrated right now. It's tough when something doesn't come easily, especially when you've been working hard on it. Let's take a break and tackle it together when you're ready." This response recognizes their emotions, normalizes their frustration, and offers support without dismissing their feelings.

It's critical to avoid judgment or blame. Resist the urge to fix or minimize their emotions right away. Acknowledge their perspective first. Here are examples of statements that validate children's feelings and experiences:

- "I can see that you're upset right now."
- "It's okay to feel sad—it's a tough situation."
- "I can tell this means a lot to you."
- "You seem frustrated about this."
- "It sounds like you're disappointed because things didn't go as planned."
- "You look like you're feeling nervous. Want to talk about it?"
- "It's normal to feel this way when something hard happens."
- "Many people would feel the same way in your situation."
- "It makes sense that you're feeling overwhelmed—it's a big deal."
- "That sounds like it was tough for you."
- "I can imagine how hurtful that must have been."
- "It must feel so disappointing when things don't turn out how you hoped."
- "I understand why you're feeling this way."
- "I get it—what happened was unfair."
- "It's okay to feel angry about this."
- "It's okay to cry if you need to."
- "Your feelings are important, and I'm here to listen."
- "Take your time—I want to understand how you're feeling."

Using these kinds of statements helps children feel seen, heard, and supported. Validation will open the door to deeper, more meaningful, and calm conversations. It also strengthens an emotional connection, showing your child that their feelings matter to you.

Asking Reflective Questions

This type of communication further deepens relationships. It involves asking open-ended, in-depth questions that prompt children to explore their thoughts, emotions, and experiences in greater detail. This way, you can encourage them to think introspectively and express themselves more deeply.

Ask a question that will spark an explanation, not just a simple yes or no answer (open-ended questions). Instead of causing an abrupt end to the dialogue, this technique invites elaboration and exploration. Here are some examples:

- "What do you think made you feel this way?"
- "How did that experience affect you?"
- "What options do you think you have?"
- "What outcome would you like to see, and why?"
- "What worked well in the past when you faced a similar situation?"
- "What could you do differently next time?"
- "How do you think the other person felt in that situation?"
- "What could you say or do to help improve your connection with them?"

The benefits of this approach are numerous. Reflective questions help children consider perspectives other than their own, which is empathy in action. They help them identify patterns in their behavior (insight) and learn from positive and negative experiences. They also encourage them to take ownership of their problems, not dwell on the negative, and find solutions.

Family Meetings

Implementing family meetings will dramatically improve communication and cohesion within any family. They allow everyone, from the youngest to the oldest, to share their thoughts and contribute to decision-making. This collaboration strengthens family bonds and teaches children indispensable skills like problem-solving and teamwork. As each person brings their unique perspective, the family becomes a more synergistic unit that learns and grows together. Regular family meetings reinforce a sense of belonging, reminding each member that they are part of something greater.

A structured approach is essential to conducting family meetings effectively. Begin by setting a regular schedule to establish consistency. Create an agenda to guide the discussion, ensuring everyone knows what to expect. Rotate leadership roles, allowing each family member to take turns facilitating the meeting. This practice empowers children, giving them a sense of responsibility and leadership.

Here is a sample family meeting agenda:

1. Compliments and/or gratitude: Each member shares something they appreciate about another member. Alternatively, each person may express gratitude for a recent positive experience.
2. Sharing the "highs and lows" of the week: This element provides insights into each person's experiences and emotions.
3. Review of previous action items: Discuss tasks or decisions from the last meeting, assess progress, and address any challenges encountered.
4. Calendar and scheduling: Review upcoming events, appointments, and activities for the week or month to keep everyone informed and prepared.
5. Open floor for concerns and suggestions: Provide a space for family members to voice concerns, propose ideas, or discuss any issues they wish to address.
6. Problem-solving: Address any issues and work together to find solutions. Assign responsibilities as needed.
7. Family activities: Discuss and plan upcoming activities or outings, ensuring everyone's interests and schedules are considered.
8. Assign chores: Review and delegate household responsibilities for the upcoming period. Ensure tasks are distributed fairly.
9. Closing remarks and next meeting: Summarize the key points discussed, confirm any decisions made, and set the date and time for the next family meeting.

As meetings progress, you'll find that they address immediate concerns and prevent many misunderstandings and arguments. Over time, these gatherings become a cherished tradition when the family comes together to listen, learn, and grow. The skills acquired during these meetings extend beyond the family, equipping children with the tools to handle social interactions and impediments in the wider world.

Relationship with Technology

In today's digital age, managing your children's relationship with technology has become a compulsory aspect of parenting. Technology offers both possibilities and difficulties. It provides incredible opportunities for learning, creativity, and connection.

However the constant presence of gadgets and screens exposes children to digital stimuli and simulated, non-real-world environments. Balancing these elements is key to raising courageous children who are deeply connected to the real world and the people around them. By managing its use thoughtfully, you can ensure technology enhances rather than hinders your children's development.

You must keep your children safe while using online platforms. The internet offers vast opportunities, but it also poses risks, such as exposure to inappropriate content, cyberbullying, online predators, scams and privacy breaches. Here are some considerations to help ensure your children's safety online.

Building trust and maintaining an open dialogue about your children's online activities is vital in ensuring their safety. When they can share their concerns or experiences without fear of judgment or punishment, they are more likely to seek guidance when needed. Ask them about the websites they visit, the apps they use, and the people they interact with online. Encourage them to talk about anything that makes them uncomfortable, reinforcing a safe and supportive environment for communication.

Educating them about online risks helps them make informed choices. They must understand the dangers of sharing personal information, clicking on unknown links, or downloading files from suspicious sources. Teaching them about scams, fake profiles, and illegitimate platforms equips them with the knowledge to negotiate the internet more safely and responsibly.

Using parental controls and monitoring apps is another effective way to safeguard your children's online activity. These tools can filter inappropriate content, set time limits, and provide oversight of permissions and settings. Regularly reviewing these limits ensures their online experience remains safe and age-appropriate.

Ensure your banking/payment information is never automatically saved on their devices. Also take care to keep your own device secure from little fingers who might not realize what they are clicking on and inadvertently purchase something unwanted or unintended.

Protecting personal information is also a principal aspect of online safety. Teach your children to use strong passwords, avoid sharing private details like their address or school, and log out of accounts when they are done. Safeguarding personal data reduces the risk of identity theft and misuse, providing them an added layer of security as they use the internet and social media.

Playing games, watching videos, or exploring websites together helps you understand their digital world. This shared involvement allows you to monitor their behavior and guide them toward safer practices.

Creating a Family Media Plan

This can be a practical step towards managing screen time effectively for the whole family. The plan can:

- Outline acceptable screen time amounts.
- The content each person can and cannot access.
- Establish screen-free zones, such as the dinner table or bedrooms.
- Designate screen-free times each day to allow time for other activities.

Establishing these clear guidelines will go a long way to helping children understand acceptable and safe behavior online, as well as control over time spent and content digested.

Modeling healthy screen habits yourself is key. Children often mimic their parents, so setting personal screen limits can be an influential example. Show them the value of unplugging by participating in offline activities together. For instance, some families establish tech-free dinner times, where everyone can share their day without digital interruptions. This practice strengthens family bonds and encourages meaningful conversations.

Scheduling a family-wide digital detox day can also offer a reprieve from the relentless pace of online life. Pre-planned tech-free days allow children to reconnect with the physical world and reduce reliance on digital validation. These breaks can realign priorities and reduce stress. Planning outdoor activities or encouraging hobbies like reading or painting also diverts attention from screens, boosting physical health and mental relaxation. By embracing these strategies, families can maintain a balanced relationship with technology.

Summary

For children, connection to their nuclear family forms the core of resilience.

A strong bond with one or more adults is required for them to mature emotionally, cognitively, and socially.

Trust, stability, and consistency underpin these connections, laying the groundwork for children to explore their world confidently.

Communication remains the lifeblood of these relationships, ensuring that every voice is heard and valued.

Chapter Three

Emotions and Empathy

Emotional Intelligence (EI), also known as Emotional Quotient (EQ), is the ability to recognize, understand, and manage one's emotions while also being able to identify, understand, and influence the feelings of others. It is a key component of effective interpersonal communication, personal development, and leadership. (Beldoch, 1964; Salovey & Mayer, 1990; Goleman, 1995). The elements to be considered are self-awareness, emotional vocabulary, emotional expression, self-regulation, and empathy. Together these components contribute to personal and professional well-being and social competence.

A robust emotional foundation equips children with healthy coping mechanisms and helps them to manage emotions during crises. This skill set also enhances their ability to form meaningful relationships as they learn to negotiate social situations.

Emotional intelligence correlates highly with academic and social success. Children who understand and regulate their emotions are better equipped to focus, solve problems, and collaborate with peers. Enhanced conflict resolution and improved stress management are natural outcomes of Emotional Intelligence, allowing children to face hardship with strength and composure.

Reflection Exercise

Are my children able to identify and articulate their emotions?

Are they able to control impulsive behaviors and delay gratification?

Do they express their feelings in healthy ways?

Can they manage strong or negative emotions?

How do they respond to seeing someone sad or in distress?

Do they adjust their behavior based on how someone is feeling?

Do they apologize and/or show regret when they hurt someone?

Emotional Awareness

Managing difficult emotions begins with the ability to recognize them when they are occurring. This is accomplished by answering these three questions:

1. What am I feeling?
2. Why am I feeling this way?
3. Are there other factors influencing my emotions?

Be sure to help them evaluate both positive and negative emotions in not only in calm situations but tense ones as well. This helps the practice to become comfortable and conditioned. Eventually, with repetition, children can identify their feelings across different contexts, uncover patterns or themes, and learn to distinguish between similar, confusing, or conflicting emotions.

Activities to Develop Emotional Awareness

Technology can be a medium for teaching soft skills in engaging and accessible ways. Many apps, games, and online resources for all ages highlight various Emotional Intelligence-building themes. By directing them towards these types of platforms, you can turn the time they spend online into something more productive.

Suggestions for pre-schoolers include:

Color your feelings: Give your children a blank outline of a body and ask them to use colors and markings to show where and how they feel emotions (e.g., red for anger, blue for sadness). Have them describe what they feel in those body parts. Examples: "Do you feel tightness in your chest when you're angry?" "Does your stomach feel fluttery when you're excited?" "Do your shoulders feel heavy when you're sad?" This will teach them to connect physical sensations with emotions.

Feelings weather report: Use weather metaphors to describe emotions. For example, "Are you feeling sunny, cloudy, or stormy today?" This will simplify emotional expression and make it fun to share their feelings.

Mood poster: Use a poster with color-coded zones to help children identify and communicate their emotional state. If they cannot articulate their feelings, they can point to a color.

Suggestions for school-age children:

Mood tracker: Create a weekly chart for children to color or mark their mood daily. Reflect on the patterns together and discuss ways to handle difficult emotions.

Daily feelings check-in: Start or end the day by asking, "How are you feeling today?" This encourages daily reflection and helps children build a habit of identifying and labeling their emotions.

Emotion drawing or writing: Ask your children to draw or write about how they feel today. Provide prompts like, "What made you happy today?" or "What was hard about today?" This encourages children to process and express emotions creatively.

Feelings jar: Keep a jar and slips of paper in a convenient location. Ask your children to write or draw how they feel each day and put it in the jar. Review the jar together at the end of the week. This promotes consistent emotional reflection and enables discussion of patterns or changes.

Feeling scales: Create a simple scale (1-10) for emotions like happiness, sadness, or anger. Ask, "On a scale of 1 to 10, how happy are you feeling right now?" This helps children to think about the intensity of their feelings and builds self-regulation skills in the process.

Gratitude and challenges check-in: At dinner or bedtime, ask, "What was the best part of your day?" and "What made you feel upset or frustrated?" This encourages self-awareness by reflecting on positive and negative emotional experiences.

Tweens might benefit from the following activities:

The body scan: This mindfulness practice concentrates on one different area of the body at a time and noticing what is felt there. It helps connect bodily sensations with emotional states. Many websites and apps offer free guided body scans, which your children can repeatedly return to.

Encourage them to keep a journal or diary to reflect on their experiences and emotions. Writing provides a cathartic outlet, allowing them to explore their thoughts more deeply and expand their emotional vocabulary. This safe space advances emotional processing and helps them better understand themselves.

Art journaling: Provide materials for drawing, painting, or collage to express their emotions visually. Use prompts like "Draw what happiness looks like to you" or "Create an image of a stressful day."

Emotion mapping: Have your children map out situations that trigger specific emotions (e.g., fear before a test, joy during a hobby). Introduce more complex feelings and discuss how different emotions can overlap (e.g., nervous and excited).

Emotional Vocabulary

Expanding children's emotional vocabulary is like giving them a map to traverse the complex terrain of their emotions. With the right words, they can articulate their feelings more clearly, which helps others understand them better. This ability reduces frustration and minimizes misunderstandings, contributing to healthier communication and emotional maturation.

Activities to Develop Emotional Vocabulary

For all ages:

A feelings wheel can help children identify and be more specific in naming their emotions. The inner circle contains basic emotions such as joy, anger, fear, sadness, disgust, or surprise. The middle circle (if present) breaks these core emotions into more detailed categories, such as anger turning into frustration or annoyance. The outer circle expands on these categories, offering more specific emotions or nuances, such as exasperation or resentment stemming from anger.

To help children use a feelings wheel, have them identify the general emotion they are experiencing (inner circle). Next, refine the feeling by looking outward on the wheel for a more specific descriptor, such as loneliness or disappointment for sadness. Repeat this process for however many circles there are on the wheel. Help your children reflect on the causes of the emotion, considering both internal and external triggers.

Different versions are available for each age group of children; wheels for younger children would have fewer and simpler emotions, while wheels for older children would have more and increasingly complex options. Consider incorporating a feelings wheel into daily routines by placing a chart on the fridge or in their room. Encourage your children to check in with their emotions at different times of the day, using the chart to articulate their feelings.

Other recommendations for preschoolers:

Mirror exercises can help them connect facial expressions with emotions, making abstract feelings more tangible. Have them look in a mirror and ask, "Can you show me how your face looks when you're happy or sad?"

Emotion face paper plates: Draw various facial expressions on paper plates. This will help children recognize different emotions and introduce more complex emotions they might not yet be familiar with.

Get a deck of flashcards with facial expressions (happy, sad, angry, etc.) and ask your children to identify or mimic the emotion. Pair emotions with real-life scenarios by laying out the flashcards and asking them, "Which card shows how you feel when you can't find your toy?"

Read books about emotions and discuss how the characters feel. Encourage children to share similar experiences.

Make a feelings collage: Provide magazines and let children cut out pictures of people showing different emotions. Discuss each element and when, where, and why they might feel those emotions.

Songs and games: Sing songs like "If You're Happy and You Know It," adding verses for other emotions (sad, scared, etc.).

School-age children may enjoy any of the above activities as well as:

Emotion dice: Make or buy a set of dice with emotion words (or faces) on each side. Roll the dice and have your children describe a time they felt that way or act it out. This makes exploring different emotions interactive and fun.

Feelings charades: Write emotions like "happy," "sad," "angry," or "excited" on slips of paper. Take turns acting out the emotion without words while others guess. This reinforces the recognition of emotions and their expressions in a fun, interactive way.

Tweens require a different approach:

Vocabulary expansion: Create a list of complex emotions (e.g., anxious, grateful, overwhelmed, disgusted, betrayed, grief) and discuss their meanings. Challenge them to use these words in conversations or writing.

Media analysis: Watch a movie or show together and discuss the characters' emotions. Ask, "Why do you think they felt that way?" and "What would you do in their situation?" This will encourage empathy and logical analysis of emotions in different contexts.

Emotions debate: Present two emotions (e.g., nervous and excited, frustrated and disappointed) and ask your tween to explain their similarities and differences. Encourage examples from their own lives.

This will deepen their understanding of emotional nuances and sharpen their communication skills.

Emotional Expression

Expressing emotions through words, actions, or behavior significantly benefits mental and physical well-being. Suppressed emotions lead to increased tension and a higher risk of mental health issues, such as depression or anxiety. Sharing feelings helps alleviate stress by providing a healthy outlet and preventing the buildup of suppressed emotions.

Within interpersonal relationships, sharing emotions supports more transparent communication, helping understand one another's needs, boundaries, and experiences. Emotional expression deepens bonds by encouraging vulnerability and trust in relationships. Constructive emotional expression prevents misunderstandings or resolves them more effectively.

If children learn to express their emotions—both positive and negative—they develop the tools to process complex feelings like grief, disappointment, betrayal, or trauma in healthier, more constructive ways. This enables them to overcome barriers, rebound from adversity, and move forward with greater clarity, closure, and inner strength. It will significantly enhance their long-term emotional well-being.

Activities to Improve Emotional Expression

Finding the right words to convey emotions can be tricky, especially when children are just starting with this practice. Here is a list of nonverbal ideas for emotional expression. Each suggestion is broadly applicable and you can tailor it to your children's ages.

Use toys like dolls, action figures, or stuffed animals and encourage your children to act out scenarios or emotions with them. For example, "Can you show me how your teddy bear is feeling today?" Play provides a safe space for children to project and process their emotions.

Body movement and dance: Ask your children to use their bodies to "show" how they feel. They might stomp if they're angry, twirl if they're happy, or curl up if they're sad. For example, "Can you move like your feelings?" Physical demonstration helps the release of emotions.

Facial expression and emoji cards: Provide cards with different facial expressions or emojis and ask your children to point to the one that matches how they feel. They can also mimic the expression. For example, "Which face looks like your feelings?"

Music selection: Play different music or ask your children to choose a song that matches their feelings. They can also use instruments to create sounds that express their mood. For example, "What song feels like your mood today?" Music helps convey emotions in ways words cannot.

Sensory activities: Provide materials like play-dough, sand, or water. Encourage them to mold, squish, or interact with the material based on their feelings. For example, "Use the play-dough to show how you're feeling." Sensory activities provide a calming and expressive outlet.

Journaling through symbols: Instead of writing words, ask your children to use symbols, shapes, or simple doodles to represent their emotions. For example, "Draw a shape that shows how big your feelings are today." It will help to organize their emotions creatively without relying on language.

Engaging in theater or drama workshops: This provides a chance to explore and express emotions through characters and storytelling. It enhances emotional expression and stimulates empathy and understanding as participants step into the shoes of others.

Writing poetry or lyrics: A cathartic form of self-expression that will allow your children to explore and communicate their emotions in a safe and creative space.

Regulation and Self-Control

Emotional regulation is the ability to manage and respond to emotions in a healthy way. It's a cornerstone of resilience, equipping children to face life's frustrations without losing composure or shutting down. When children can regulate their emotions, they gain control over their behavior, leading to better interactions. It will also maintain their ability to focus, learn, and engage positively with their environment, even during times of provocation.

Strategies to Develop Self-Regulation

Encourage physical activity and movement: Sports, dancing, yoga, or simple workouts can help children release pent-up energy and emotions.

Impulse control games help children practice pausing before reacting. They build patience and forethought, essential skills for regulation. They also increase listening skills, following instructions, delayed gratification, and staying attentive:

- Red Light, Green Light: One person acts as the "traffic light" and calls out "green light!" (children move) or "red light!" (children freeze). If a child moves on "red light," they return to the start or pause briefly before continuing.

- Freeze Dance: Play music and encourage children to dance. When the music stops, they must freeze in place. Anyone caught moving after the music stops is out for that round.

- Simon Says: The leader gives commands prefaced by "Simon says..." (e.g., "Simon says touch your nose"). If the command is given without "Simon says," children must not follow it.

- The Marshmallow Test: Place a marshmallow (or any treat) in front of the children. Tell them they'll get two marshmallows if they wait 5 minutes without eating it.

Techniques to Manage Emotional Outbursts

You will need some tricks in your back pocket to manage the inevitable tantrums and other difficult emotions that occasionally occur. Incorporating these items into daily life can help children self-soothe and will have a preventative effect. Experiment with different approaches to determine which best supports your children's sensory and emotional needs.

Use distraction or redirection: Shift their attention to a different activity or object, such as a favorite toy or a drawing activity. Distraction can interrupt the cycle of escalating emotions and provide time to calm down.

Offer choices: To regain a sense of control, give the children two acceptable options. For example, "Would you like to draw or play with blocks to calm down?" Empowering children with choices can diffuse tension and encourage cooperation.

Create a calm-down space: Set up a specific area in your home with decreased sensory stimuli (quiet, dim lights) where your children can regain composure. This space can include comforting items like soft pillows or favorite books, providing a retreat during overwhelming moments.

Rocking chairs or swings: Rhythmic motions soothe the nervous system, similar to how rocking comforts infants.

Sensory swing/hammock: This long piece of cloth hangs from the ceiling and wraps around the body, creating a sense of security and comfort.

This "cocoon" effect can mimic deep-pressure input, known to calm the nervous system. Feeling enveloped can reduce overstimulation and help children feel grounded. Sitting or lying in a hammock encourages them to remain still and focus on their body and surroundings, promoting mindfulness.

Weighted blankets: The gentle pressure provides deep touch stimulation, calming the nervous system and reducing anxiety by releasing serotonin and melatonin (bodily substances that promote calm and happiness).

Fidget toys such as stress balls, spinners, tangle toys, or sensory rings: Engaging the hands with repetitive motions or textures helps redirect attention and reduce nervous energy.

Aromatherapy using essential oil diffusers, incense, sachets, bath bombs, or scented candles: Certain scents, like lavender or chamomile, reduce stress and promote relaxation.

Sensory bottles: Watching glitter or small objects slowly settle in a liquid-filled bottle can have a meditative and calming effect.

Chewy necklaces or gum: Chewing provides oral sensory input, which can reduce stress and help regulate emotions.

Yoga or stability balls: Sitting or lightly bouncing on a yoga ball provides calming proprioceptive input, helping to ground the body.

Sensory mats or textures: Walking barefoot on textured mats or using sensory cushions engages tactile input and can reduce anxiety.

Controlled Breathing

Guiding your children in deep breathing exercises can help them calm down during emotional distress. Breathing (especially exhalation) activates the parasympathetic nervous system, reducing stress and anxiety. It also improves focus by centering attention on one thing during overwhelming moments. Below are some simple but effective breathing exercises you can guide your children through.

Smell the Flower, Blow the Candle: Pretend to hold a flower in one hand and a candle in the other. Inhale deeply through the nose as if smelling the flower, then exhale slowly out of the mouth to blow out the candle. This technique makes breathing fun and relatable for young children while promoting slow, controlled breaths.

5-Finger Breathing: Hold one hand up with fingers spread wide. Use the other hand's index finger to trace up and down each finger while breathing. Inhale through the nose as you trace up, exhale out the mouth as you trace down. This provides a tactile fixation to keep the children engaged. Example: "Let's trace your hand like we're climbing a mountain. Breathe in as you climb up and out as you go down."

Box Breathing: Inhale through the nose for a count of four, hold the breath for four, exhale through the mouth for four, and pause for four. Visualize a square and trace its sides with each phase, then repeat as necessary.

Progressive Muscle Relaxation

A method of tensing and releasing muscles, this helps release stress and calm the mind. Here is a sample script:

Hands: "Let's start with your hands. Squeeze your hands into tight fists like you're holding two squishy balls. Squeeze as hard as you can... 1, 2, 3... and now let go. Let your hands relax. Feel how soft and loose they are now. Great!"

Arms and shoulders: "Next, pretend you're a turtle hiding in its shell. Shrug your shoulders up to your ears and pull your arms in tight like you're hiding. Hold it... 1, 2, 3... and now relax. Let your shoulders drop and feel how much lighter they are."

Face and jaw: "Now, let's move to your face. Pretend you just bit into a super sour lemon. Scrunch your face up really tight—wrinkle your nose, close your eyes, and squeeze your mouth. Hold it... 1, 2, 3... and now let your face relax. Feel how soft your cheeks and forehead are now. Good job!"

Stomach: "Now imagine you're trying to hold a big beach ball on your tummy. Squeeze your belly tight, like you're holding it in place. Hold it... 1, 2, 3... and now let go. Let your belly feel soft and relaxed."

Legs: "Let's focus on your legs now. Pretend you're squishing sand between your toes. Tighten your legs all the way from your toes to your thighs. Hold it... 1, 2, 3... and now relax. Let your legs feel heavy and loose."

Whole body: "Now, let's squeeze your whole body from your head to your toes. Pretend you're a stiff statue. Squeeze everything tight—your hands, arms, face, belly, and legs. Hold it... 1, 2, 3... and now let it all go. Let your whole body feel soft and relaxed."

Mental Health

Discussing mental health openly and regularly with your children is fundamental to a lifetime of well-being. When you make mental health a regular topic of conversation, you normalize the issue and decrease the shame and stigma that are often associated with some conditions. This will make it easier for children to seek help should they need it in the future. Use age-appropriate language to explain complex concepts.

You can describe emotions using **simple comparisons** and relatable examples. Examples include describing sadness as a gray cloud that will eventually pass and depression as feeling stuck or carrying a heavy backpack. Anxiety could be described as butterflies in their stomach. Or you might say, "Anxiety is like having a worry that doesn't go away, even when there's nothing to be afraid of. It's like your brain is trying to protect you from danger, but sometimes it gets confused and makes you feel scared or nervous when everything is actually okay." These metaphors help children grasp feelings they may not understand.

As they grow, introduce more detailed explanations. A description of depression might sound like, "Sometimes, people feel really sad or tired for a long time, even when nothing bad is happening. This is called depression. It's like having a heavy cloud over your head that makes everything feel harder, even things you usually enjoy. It can make people feel like they don't have energy, want to be alone, or are stuck in a bad mood, and can't get out of it. But there is help for depression to make that heavy feeling go away."

Emphasize that it's **okay to talk about feelings** and encourage them to ask for help, reassuring them that there are ways to feel better. It's also beneficial to emphasize hope, explaining that depression isn't permanent and that with support, like engaging in therapy, those heavy feelings can lift. This approach makes the conversation accessible and reassuring for children.

Highlight to your children that **mental health is as important as physical health**. Your explanation might sound like this, "Just like we take care of our bodies by eating healthy foods, getting enough sleep, and exercising, we also need to take care of our minds. When we feel sad, scared, or worried, our brain needs extra help, like when we might need a bandage for a cut or medicine for a cold. Taking care of our mental health can mean talking about our feelings, asking for help when we need it, or doing things that make us feel calm and happy. A healthy mind helps us feel better, learn new things, and enjoy life fully."

Discuss the impact of mental health on daily life, ensuring they understand that mental health affects how we think, feel, and act. Share your personal experiences, if appropriate, to normalize these conversations. For instance, talking about how you felt anxious before a big meeting can help your children relate and understand that these feelings are normal and manageable. By having these dialogues, you create a household that openly acknowledges and values mental health, building a foundation for lifelong well-being.

Technology and Emotional Well-Being

In today's connected world, technology is a constant companion for children. While it offers endless opportunities for learning and communication, it can also affect their emotional well-being. Here are a few of the dynamics to be aware of.

The constant connectivity creates a sense of urgency, leading to anxiety as children feel pressured to respond instantly to messages and notifications. This barrage of notifications also causes incessant distractions that impair focus and productivity. The addicting nature of constant notifications can make it hard for children to disconnect. This relentless pace can overwhelm them, leaving little room for reflection or relaxation.

Social media offers a platform for individuals to express themselves, connect with others, and explore new ideas. Yet, its very nature can profoundly affect self-esteem and mental health. Imagine scrolling through endless photos and updates that paint a perfect picture of other people's lives. This façade is misleading, as we know that social media often presents a highly edited version of reality, where peers look better, appear happier, more successful, or more socially active than they may be. Many children feel compelled to match these idealized portrayals.

It's easy for children to feel envious. This comparison culture can erode self-esteem as children measure themselves against carefully manufactured images of peers. These comparisons can lead to feelings of inadequacy, impacting their self-worth when their lives don't seem to measure up.

The constant need for social acceptance in virtual communities adds another layer of pressure. The quest for "likes" and "followers" has become a status symbol. Children question their worth if they don't get the attention they crave or feel they deserve.

Compounding this is the "fear of missing out" (FOMO), a feeling of exclusion or sadness that arises when children believe they are being left out of fun or meaningful experiences that others are participating in. This fear or disappointment of exclusion can significantly impact mental well-being, often leading to increased levels of anxiety, depression, and low self-esteem.

Mitigation Strategies

Build a supportive network: Help your children surround themselves with friends and peers who value authenticity over appearances. Positive social circles will reduce the pressure on them to conform to unrealistic standards. Face-to-face relationships will provide genuine emotional support. Prioritize in-person activities with friends and family, such as sports or hobbies. Real-world interactions provide meaningful connections, reducing the need to seek validation through social media.

Encourage diverse interests: Motivate your children to explore hobbies and activities that don't rely on social media, such as sports, art, or volunteering. Pursuing offline passions builds friendships and provides fulfillment outside of the digital world.

Help children understand that social media often presents an idealized version of life: People tend to share only their happiest moments, successes, or carefully revised images. Many positive posts are edited, staged, or filtered to appear perfect. They rarely reflect the complete picture of someone's life. Negative experiences and emotions are seldom posted. For example, a smiling photo might not show the difficult moments before or after, or a glamorous vacation post might be more about impressing others than genuine enjoyment.

By pointing this out, you can teach children to approach social media skeptically, recognizing that what they see online isn't always the truth. This builds a critical perspective. It will help them to separate online portrayals from reality, reducing the impact of unrealistic comparisons.

Discussing FOMO honestly with your children helps them understand it's a normal and shared experience. Explain that everyone, including adults, sometimes feels left out or wishes to be part of something they see others doing. It doesn't define their worth or happiness.

Stress that they remain valued and loved despite missing a particular event. You can also emphasize the benefits of taking breaks from constant social engagement, such as having time to recharge, develop personal interests, or connect more deeply with close friends and family.

Explain that while feelings of FOMO can feel intense in the moment, they often pass and don't mean they're truly missing out on anything meaningful. Share your experiences with FOMO, such as feeling disappointed about not being invited to a party or seeing friends on a trip you couldn't attend.

Encourage them to reflect on past enjoyable experiences. Helping children build this perspective equips them with the tools to manage FOMO without feeling overwhelmed or pressured into constantly comparing themselves to others.

Empathy

Empathy is the ability to understand and share another person's feelings, experiences, or perspectives. It involves recognizing what someone else is going through emotionally and mentally and imagining how it might feel to be in their situation.

Empathy allows us to connect with others on a deeper level, encouraging compassion and kindness. Viewing an experience from someone else's perspective facilitates better support of that individual. It also enables one to form an appropriate response that shows care and understanding. It's a foundational skill for building healthy relationships and creating community.

Empathy is a combination of innate tendencies and learned behaviors. Humans are born with the basic capacity for empathy, as evidenced by babies crying when they hear another baby cry. However, parenting, social interactions, and cultural norms shape how people express empathy.

Strategies to Encourage Empathy

One of the most effective ways to teach empathy is by **modeling it yourself**. Children emulate their parents' behaviors, so they will naturally adopt similar behaviors when they see you showing compassion and understanding toward others.

Regularly **acknowledging and addressing others' feelings** through your actions and words can reinforce this. For example, "That boy looks sad; let's ask if he's okay," or "That person seems to be struggling with their groceries; let's help them."

Make **sharing and taking turns** mandatory: Engage in games and activities that involve sharing to generate awareness of others' needs. For example, "Let's make sure everyone gets a turn with the crayons."

Encourage **acts of kindness**, such as helping with chores or writing thank-you notes. These actions build an understanding of others' needs and feelings. For example, "Your sister is feeling sad. Maybe giving her a hug would help."

Promote **perspective-taking**: Prompt your children to imagine how others might feel in different situations. For example, "How do you think your friend felt when they weren't picked for the team?"

Praise **empathetic behavior**: Recognize and affirm moments when your children show empathy or kindness. For example, "It was so thoughtful of you to share your snack with your friend who forgot theirs."

Expose them to **diversity**: Create opportunities to learn about different cultures, experiences, or people facing barriers. Read books about different lifestyles and traditions. Eat at a restaurant with food different from your own culture. Get them involved in community service or helping others in need, like donating clothes or volunteering at an animal shelter.

Try the "**Walk a Mile in Their Shoes**" activity:

- Gather a few pairs of shoes or create character cards representing different people, situations, or experiences. Examples include a new child at school, someone who has lost a favorite toy, or someone nervous about speaking in front of a crowd.

- Place the shoes or cards in a line. Explain that each pair of shoes or card represents a different person and their unique situation or feelings.

- Invite them to choose a pair of shoes or a card. Ask them to step into the shoes, literally or figuratively, and imagine what it's like to be that person. Prompt: "Imagine you are [person]. What might you be feeling?" "What problems might you face?" "How would you want others to treat you?"

- Afterward, discuss their observations and realizations. Questions might include, "How did it feel to be in their shoes?" "What might help this person feel better?" "What can we do to be kind or supportive of someone in this situation?"

Summary

Emotional Intelligence plays a pivotal role in building resilience. Identifying and managing emotions lays solid ground for handling life's challenges.

By expanding their emotional vocabulary, children gain the language required to articulate their feelings, reducing miscommunication and forming deeper connections.

Emotional regulation is a consequential skill for maintaining composure in times of stress. Empathy is the cornerstone of social development, teaching children to see the world through others' eyes.

Together, these components form a comprehensive framework for advancing emotional well-being and equipping children with the tools they need to thrive as individuals and in relationships.

Chapter Four

Growth Mindset

Adopting a growth mindset as a parent can transform your family dynamic and your approach to difficulties. When you implement this mindset, you show your children that learning and improvement are lifelong endeavors. This shift in perspective can make a world of difference, creating an environment where children feel safe to explore and make mistakes. Embedded within in this paradigm are curiosity and motivation, which are imperative for lifelong success. By embracing flexibility and optimism, you will not only instill these traits in your children, but also learn to adapt to new parenting dilemmas as your children get older.

What is a Growth Mindset?

Psychologist Carol Dweck coined the term to describe the belief that talents and intelligence are modifiable traits developed through dedication and hard work (2006). This perspective contrasts with the fixed mindset, in which people view abilities as unchangeable. A growth mindset reframes troubles as opportunities to learn and improve rather than obstacles to avoid.

Children who believe in their ability to improve are more likely to persevere, even when faced with difficulties. This determination is essential to tackle life's hurdles that will eventually come their way. A growth mindset shifts the emphasis from seeing failure as an endpoint to valuing learning and self-advancement.

Children with this perspective understand that effort leads to progress and are more motivated to keep trying, even when encountering setbacks. This outlook encourages them to try new things without fear of failure, fostering openness to challenge and a willingness to explore new experiences.

Introducing growth mindset principles early in childhood can profoundly shape a child's approach to learning and problem-solving. Young children, naturally inquisitive and eager to explore, benefit significantly from encouragement that reinforces their curiosity. Through your encouragement, they develop belief in their abilities and build foundational problem-solving skills, setting the stage for a lifelong love of learning.

A growth mindset enhances openness to new experiences. By teaching children to approach challenges with curiosity and a willingness to experiment, you help them develop tenacity and adaptability, equipping them to succeed in a world full of possibilities.

Reflection Exercise

What type of praise do I offer my children?

Am I patient with the learning process?

Do I allow my children time to find solutions, or do I intervene quickly?

How do I respond to my children's mistakes?

How do I respond when my children say, "I can't do this"?

How do I handle adversity in my life?

Am I modeling a willingness to learn and improve in front of my children?

What is something about myself I've been wanting to change?

Has a fixed mindset prevented me from doing this?

How to Adopt a Growth Mindset

The language used when interacting with children is imperative to fostering a growth mindset. Positive reinforcement and constructive feedback teach them that effort leads to progress. Instead of praising innate talent—such as saying, "You're so smart," — point to their *efforts*, e.g., "I'm proud of how hard you worked on this." This subtle but impactful shift emphasizes that betterment is achievable through diligence and effort.

Here are some other ways to develop a Growth Mindset:

- "Mistake of the Day" reflection, where they discuss a mistake and what they learned from it.
- Create an atmosphere where there is no such thing as a dumb question.

- Academically, change the focus from high grades to viewing exams as learning opportunities, always with room for improvement.
- During extracurricular activities, emphasize skill development, collaboration, and perseverance rather than winning.

These suggestions are from Sara Briggs (2015):

- Accept and embrace your children's flaws. Avoiding weaknesses makes it impossible to overcome them.
- Replace the word "failing" with "learning." Every mistake or unmet goal is a chance to learn, not a failure.
- Prioritize the journey over the outcome.
- Experiment with various methods of learning (see Chapter 2).
- Redefine what it means to be smart. True intelligence requires dedication and effort, not talent alone.
- Incorporate the word "yet" into your children's vocabulary. For example, "I'm no good at this.....yet."
- Gain insights from others' mistakes. Everyone shares common struggles, which can serve as valuable lessons.
- Prioritize progression over speed. Mastering a skill thoroughly takes time.
- View the brain as a muscle that needs exercise and practice to get good at something, just like every other muscle in the body.
- Maintain a long-term perspective by keeping the larger goal in sight.
- Deter your children from seeking your or anyone else's approval. Fixating on someone else's goals will hinder their inherent ability to progress.
- Set a new goal for every goal they achieve. Remember, the journey of learning is never-ending.

Curiosity

Curiosity is a powerful force for learning and innovation. It is the spark that fuels discovery and cognitive development. It motivates children to explore their environment, ask questions, and seek greater understanding. This natural curiosity forms the foundation for a lifelong passion for learning, driving them to approach new topics with enthusiasm and eagerness.

Through exploration, children develop essential problem-solving skills and learn the value of trial and error. This process encourages critical and adaptive thinking, equipping them with valuable tools to succeed in an ever-changing world. Curiosity facilitates knowledge acquisition and promotes an innovative mindset. With curiosity, children can tackle evolving problems with fresh perspectives and creative solutions.

Your role in modeling curiosity is incredibly important. Children learn by watching those around them, and your behavior significantly influences their desire to explore. When you show curiosity in everyday activities, you set an example, encouraging your children to ask questions and seek new experiences.

Show enthusiasm for learning new things, whether reading a book on a topic you've never explored or experimenting with a new recipe. Share your discoveries with your children, discussing the joy of uncovering something new. This behavior nurtures their inquisitiveness and reinforces learning as a lifelong pursuit.

Nurturing Curiosity

Creating a stimulating home environment rich with diverse materials is key. Fill their space with books, puzzles, art supplies, and interactive toys that invite exploration and learning.

Give your children opportunities to explore through hands-on activities like science experiments, gardening, cooking, or building. Engaging their senses and involving them in active discovery sparks interest and creativity. For example, "Let's plant these seeds and see what happens. How do you think they'll grow?"

Foster a culture where your children feel safe to ask questions, even if you don't have the answers. Respond with interest and encourage further exploration. For example, "That's a great question! What do you think the answer might be? Let's look it up together!"

Learn together by visiting museums, parks, or nature trails. Experiencing the world firsthand stimulates investigation and inspires questions. For example, "Look at this exhibit about space. What do you think astronauts eat in space?"

Motivation

Building intrinsic motivation and self-drive in children is necessary for their long-term accomplishments. These traits empower them to pursue goals with passion and tenacity, teaching them to overcome setbacks with determination. Children who are internally driven engage in activities because they find them rewarding, not because they feel pressured or expect external rewards. This inner desire to learn and advance instills a love for discovery that supports perseverance and adaptability in facing life's quandaries.

Reflection Exercise

What activities do my children engage in enthusiastically?

Do they rely on external rewards to complete tasks?

Do they put consistent effort into activities they care about?

How do my children approach tasks they find less enjoyable?

What do teachers or coaches say about their engagement and effort?

What drives me to pursue my current goals?

Am I motivated by internal desires or external pressures?

What strategies do I use to maintain motivation during difficult times?

Increasing Motivation

Take the time to understand **what excites and interests your children** by observing their natural inclinations and passions. Encourage them toward activities and subjects they genuinely enjoy and feel curious about, as this can fuel their intrinsic motivation. Allow them the freedom to explore different hobbies and experiences so they can uncover what truly inspires and fulfills them. You help them build a sense of purpose by supporting their interests.

Positive reinforcement is a formidable tool in boosting motivation. Praise for effort and perseverance creates a supportive environment where children feel encouraged to push their limits. When feedback is required, make sure it is constructive. Focus on specific elements rather than criticizing the failure as a whole. This helps children understand the specific areas needing improvement.

Here are some other simple but effective ways to spark motivation in your children:

- Offer a reward for games and activities (e.g., a scavenger hunt). The reward reinforces the joy of completing a task, encouraging a positive cycle of effort and achievement.

- Create a personal or family mission statement or a mantra that reflects their aspirations.

- Share your stories of ambition and success with them.

- Read books and watch documentaries about people who became successful through motivation and hard work. This will stimulate internal dialogue that says, "If they can do it, I can do it, too."

- Celebrate milestones and victories. By celebrating, you show them that you value and notice their hard work. This recognition fuels their drive to continue pushing forward, even when they face difficulties.

Optimism

A positive outlook isn't about ignoring problems or pretending everything is perfect. It's about emphasizing solutions instead of barriers and the good that prevails in difficult situations. Optimism provides a buffer during tough times, allowing children to maintain motivation despite adversity. They learn to view each setback as a stepping stone rather than a stumbling block. Over time, they will become better equipped to handle life's ups and downs.

Adopting a positive outlook has many benefits. It produces higher levels of happiness and life satisfaction and reduces the risk of depression. Optimistic individuals have stronger immune systems, enhancing their ability to fight illnesses. They also live longer because of healthier lifestyles and lower stress levels.

Optimism plays a key role in improving relationships by fostering empathy, understanding, and support. It enhances communication by promoting constructive conversations, reducing conflicts, and minimizing misunderstandings. Positive individuals attract others with similar energy, building a strong, supportive network.

Professionally, optimism boosts work performance by encouraging productivity, proactivity, and strength under pressure. Idealist leaders inspire and motivate their teams more effectively, which drives success and company profits. A positive outlook also helps students stay motivated, manage stress, and achieve better outcomes.

Strategies To Adopt Optimism

You can learn and adopt a positive mindset as a conscious choice. Deliberate effort and practice are required, but like any muscle in the body, when exercised, the optimism muscle will eventually become stronger and more accessible. Here are just a few ideas to practice with your children:

- Practice gratitude: Help them name or write three things they're grateful for daily.
- Express appreciation: Remind them to thank people for their kindness or support.
- Surround them with uplifting and encouraging people; Distance them from people or situations that are consistently negative.
- Fill their space with things that bring them joy, such as inspiring books, art, or music.
- Replace their pessimistic thoughts or words with constructive alternatives.
- Focus on solutions: When problems arise, determine what you and they can do about them rather than dwelling on the negative.
- Get them engaging in acts of kindness by volunteering, complimenting someone, or lending a hand.
- Help them pursue activities that bring them joy.
- Limit exposure to the news and social media (these platforms tend towards fear and pessimistic storylines).
- Have them visualize success: Help them frequently imagine and discuss their desired outcomes.
- Affirmations: Write positive statements on small pieces of paper (or on windows or mirrors) and place them around the house. Get them to stand in front of the mirror and speak these statements to themselves and affirm their ability to achieve their goals. Eventually, they will incorporate these beliefs into their subconscious mind.

Goal Setting

Goal setting is like charting a course on a map—it provides direction and purpose to life's journey. It gives children a sense of control, empowering them to take ownership of their growth. By establishing clear goals, children learn to channel their efforts effectively, track their progress, and celebrate their achievements, increasing self-efficacy and motivation.

Short-term goals provide quick wins, keeping your children's stimulus high. These might include completing a book or finishing a project. Long-term goals, like saving for a desired toy or improving in a sport, teach patience and perseverance. Both goals work together, helping children see the connection between effort and achievement. This practice builds endurance and a proactive mindset, encouraging children to take initiative in their learning and development.

Start by asking your children **what they want** to achieve in school, sports, or other activities. Then, to make goal setting more effective, follow the SMART framework: Specific, Measurable, Achievable, Relevant, and Time-Bound. This approach provides clarity, ensuring goals are realistic and attainable.

Help them **track progress** creatively using charts, journals, or digital apps. Visual reminders, like a colorful poster on the fridge, keep goals in the forefront. This will also cue the timing of celebrating achievements.

While setting ambitious goals is exciting, avoiding unrealistic expectations is also imperative. Helping your children understand their limits prevents discouragement and fosters a healthy perspective on progress. Encourage your children to stretch themselves, but remind them that setbacks are part of the process.

You should also set some goals for your own personal or professional development. As you strive for continuous improvement, you inspire your children to do the same. Perhaps you've always wanted to learn a new skill or overcome a personal hurdle. Share this journey with your children, discussing your efforts, setbacks, and triumphs. This transparency strengthens your bond and shows the value of perseverance.

Also, consider **setting goals as a family**, like planning a vacation or volunteering together. These shared objectives teach children the value of collaboration and collective effort. By working toward common goals, families create a supportive environment where everyone feels valued and inspired.

Summary

A growth mindset teaches children to see challenges as potential for improvement rather than insurmountable obstacles.

Children learn to persevere by embracing mistakes and concentrating on effort. You can cultivate this mindset through deliberate actions and language.

You play a crucial role in modeling this mindset, showing your children how to approach life's hurdles with curiosity, motivation, and optimism.

Chapter Five

Thinking, Solving and Deciding

The fast pace of today's world makes the ability to think critically, solve problems, and make sound decisions an essential life skill. The essence of thinking lies in the ability to analyze situations, weigh options, and foresee consequences. Solving is about applying this knowledge to find practical and effective solutions to problems. Decision-making, the final piece of the puzzle, involves choosing a path forward, often amidst uncertainty and competing priorities. Your role is to help your children approach each element in a practical and logical way and with a discerning eye.

Reflection Exercise

Do my children attempt to solve problems independently?

Are they calm and methodical, or do they get frustrated and give up?

Do they come up with creative solutions or rely on familiar ones?

Do they weigh the pros and cons before deciding?

Are their decisions thoughtful or impulsive?

Do I encourage them to explore different points of view?

How do I guide them in making informed decisions?

Critical Thinking

Imagine your children are facing a dilemma: They're invited to two birthday parties on the same day, both hosted by close friends. How do they decide where to go? This seemingly small decision is an opportunity to practice critical thinking, a skill that will help them navigate more complex predicaments as they mature.

Critical thinking is the ability to analyze information and make informed decisions. It involves questioning assumptions, evaluating evidence, and drawing conclusions based on facts. Emotions should not play a huge role; the logical part of the brain should take the lead. This process not only aids in everyday choices but teaches children to approach problems systematically and thoroughly. Here are several frameworks that you can choose and adapt to your children's age and abilities.

The "5 Whys" Method

To better understand a problem's root cause, ask "why" at least five times. Each time you ask "why," you dig deeper to determine the real reason behind what's happening. This approach helps avoid superficial fixes and reveals the problem's root cause for a permanent solution (Toyoda, ca. 1930s). To implement this strategy, try it on something inconsequential, such as a broken toy. If practiced and perfected in a non-threatening environment, it will become more effective for your children when the stakes are higher.

Example: Child, "I don't want to go to bed!" Parent: "You don't want to go to bed. Why not?" Child: "Because I'm not tired."

Parent: "Why do you think you're not tired?" Child: "Because I was watching TV and now I'm wide awake."

Parent: "Why do you feel wide awake after watching TV?" Child: "Because the show was really exciting."

Parent: "Why does an exciting show make it hard to sleep?" Child: "Because my brain keeps thinking about it and I can't relax."

Parent: "Why do you think your brain keeps thinking about it?" Child: "Because there was a scary part and now I keep remembering it."

Insight: The child isn't just "being defiant" — their mind is overstimulated (and even a little scared) from what they watched. Now the parent can help by offering a calm bedtime routine, turning off screens earlier in the evening or talking through any scary thoughts before bed.

"If-Then" Logic

This technique establishes a cause-and-effect relationship where a specific condition (the "if" statement) leads to a particular result (the "then" statement). It will help your children understand how actions lead to consequences and help them choose the best course of action based on expected results.

Examples: *If* you add too much water to the dough, *then* it will become sticky. *If* you don't clean up your toys, *then* you won't have time to play outside. *If* you touch something hot, *then* you might burn your hand. *If* you don't wear your jacket, *then* you might feel cold.

"Circle of Viewpoints"

This strategy encourages children to explore different perspectives other than their own. Ask them, "What might this look like from someone else's point of view?" This method promotes empathy and perspective-taking, teaching children to consider diverse viewpoints and understand the complexity of issues (Harvard Graduate School of Education, 2019).

Example: Child: "It's so unfair that teachers give homework on weekends!"

Parent: What do you think your teacher's viewpoint on this would be?" Child: "Maybe... they think we need extra practice?"

Parent: "Good! Now, what about your parents' viewpoint?" Child: "Umm... maybe they think homework keeps me busy and learning?'

Parent: "Awesome thinking. What about another student's viewpoint — maybe someone who likes homework?" Child: "Maybe they think it's easy and it helps them get better grades."

Parent: "And if you were the principal — what would your viewpoint be about weekend homework?" Child: "Maybe I'd think homework should be short so kids still have time to rest and be with family."

Concrete outcome: Instead of just venting, the child practices empathy (seeing others' perspectives), critical thinking and problem-solving (suggesting balanced solutions).

Digital Literacy

More information is readily available to humans than ever before in history. Gone are the days of opening an encyclopedia from your parent's bookshelf to write a school paper. But along with helpful information comes a plethora of misinformation and non-credible references. What sources are legitimate, and what sources should be ignored? How do children, who are more gullible than adults, learn to tell the difference?

The ability to **evaluate online content judiciously** can shape children's understanding of the world, influencing their perspectives and decisions. As a parent, you want to ensure they ingest correct and credible information. Digital literacy will transform your children from being passive consumers into informed participants. It will help them question the authenticity of online content, prompting them to think twice before accepting information as truth.

Website Credibility

Help your children understand that not everything online is true or made by experts. Some people or websites share fake stories to get attention, make money, or even confuse others. When viewing online content, they should keep the following questions in mind:

- Who is providing this information?
- When was it published or updated?
- Where is the information coming from (source credibility)?
- How was the information obtained?
- Why was it created (to inform, sell, persuade, entertain)?
- Who seeks to benefit from this information becoming widespread?

Assist them to realize there are reputable sources of information on the internet but there are non-credible sources as well. Not everyone in the world has honorable or genuine intentions with the content they produce. Tell them that not everything they see online is true or neutral, and it's important to know the difference. Let them know that if they believe everything without checking facts or sources, they might end up sharing fake stories or making choices based on lies.

You can show them that the credibility of a website can often be determined by looking at its URL. Government agencies use ". gov" websites; these are credible sources. This would apply to industrialized countries only. Likewise, if the URL ends in ". edu," it is an academic journal and can be considered credible. Warn your children to be cautious of sites with unusual domain names, excessive ads, or extensions like ".com.co" or ".biz."

Legitimate websites will look professionally designed, be fully functional (no broken links), and be easy to navigate. The content should reference other credible sources or studies. An illegitimate website may look unprofessional and messy and have spelling, grammar, and punctuation mistakes. They should be cautious of websites that use emotionally charged language, unverified claims, or lack multiple perspectives.

Teach them to check the "About Us" section. Look for the author's name and credentials. Are they an expert in the field? Is the author associated with a reputable organization or institution, such as a university? Credible sources often provide contact details or links to the author's professional profile. They also typically display editors or a review process to further prove their legitimacy. Red flags to take note of include no author, an author with no credentials, no references or citations, claims that sound too good to be true and excessive pop-up ads or clickbait headlines.

Internet Algorithms

It may also be beneficial to discuss the concept of internet algorithms with your children. You may start by mentioning that if it sometimes seems like apps "know" what type of content they like and seem to show them more of the same. This is because of algorithms.

An algorithm is like a recipe for a computer—it's a set of instructions that tells the app what to do. When your children watch videos, click on posts, or like pictures, the app "learns" what they enjoy. It uses this information to show them more things they might like, hoping that they'll spend more time on the app.

But this can lead to something called *confirmation bias*. It occurs when people only see or believe information that matches what they already think, instead of getting the truth or the full story. This can make it feel like their opinion is 100% right because they're not seeing anything that disagrees with it—even though the world is full of different opinions and facts. It presents a serious impediment to critical thinking, empathy and informed decision making.

You can explain to your children that confirmation bias can make it harder for anyone, especially children, to learn and grow. If they only see things that they agree with, they might miss out on other important ideas or facts. It's like watching only one part of a movie and thinking you know the whole story.

Therefore it's important to look at all different angles of a topic (and other people's point of view) and not let just the algorithms dictate what content is consumed. By staying curious, asking questions and examining all sides of a topic, your children can make better decisions and understand the world in a more balanced way.

Problem-Solving

Problem-solving involves recognizing a problem, gathering information to better understand the situation, thinking of solutions, and choosing the best one to try. After implementing a solution, reflection on the results determines whether it worked or if another approach would be better. This section suggests several methods to help your children develop this valuable skill.

A Problem-Solving Chart is a visual tool for breaking down complex issues into manageable steps. The chart ensures consideration of all problem aspects and potential solutions. Arrows connect shapes and colors to show the sequence of steps. The steps include mapping out the problem, potential solutions, consequences of each solution, the chosen solution, and its outcome. This tool will help your children organize their thoughts and evaluate options systematically.

The STAR Model encourages children to be mindful and reflective in problem-solving:

Stop: Pause to understand the problem.

Think: Consider potential solutions.

Act: Implement the chosen solution.

Reflect: Review the outcome and what you learned.

Example: Deciding whether to share a favorite toy with a friend. **S**top: Pause to think instead of acting out of frustration. **T**hink: Sharing could make your friend happy and help the playtime go smoothly. **A**ct: Decide to share the toy. **R**eflect: Feel good about how sharing made both of you happy.

The IDEAL Model (Bransford & Stein, 1984) provides a simple structure for children to work through any issue. The acronym makes the steps easy to remember:

Identify the problem: What is the problem that needs to be solved?

Define and represent the problem: What information is available about the situation? What actions will address the problem?

Explore feasible solutions: What can be tried to solve this problem?

Act on the chosen solution: What should be tried first?

Look back and learn: Did the plan work? What did you learn? What can be done differently next time?

Consider the following example:

Identify the problem: "I lost my homework, and I need to find it or figure out what to do before school tomorrow."

Define and represent the problem: "I know I had my homework when I left school. I might have left it in my backpack, at school, or home."

Explore possible strategies: "Recheck my backpack, look in the places I was at home (desk, kitchen, living room), and ask a parent or sibling if they've seen it. If I still can't find it, ask a classmate for the assignment details or email my teacher."

Act on the strategy: "I'll check my backpack first. If it's not there, I'll look in my room and ask my parents for help."

Look back and learn: "I found the homework under my desk. Next time, I'll put it directly in my backpack after I finish it. Lesson learned: I must organize my homework better.

Encouraging children to apply problem-solving skills creatively can be both fun and educational. For all ages, scavenger hunts offer a playful way to define what they're searching for, plan their route, and adjust strategies based on clues. Older children might enjoy escape room games, analyzing clues, solving puzzles, and collaborating with peers. It might also be possible to task your children with planning a family event within a budget. They must define the event's scope, analyze costs, propose solutions like cutting unnecessary expenses, and evaluate the results. These activities reinforce problem-solving skills and bolster creativity, collaboration, and leadership.

Decision Making

No matter how trivial it seems, each decision plays an integral role in shaping children's character and development. Making choices encourages children to exercise judgment, a skill that increases their confidence and autonomy. When children make choices, they learn about responsibility and accountability—understanding that their choices have consequences. Guiding your children through these decisions is a way to support their ability to think independently and trust themselves.

Encouraging decision-making from a young age lays the groundwork for this independence. Visual aids like charts or pictures can help preschoolers make simple choices, such as picking a snack or storybook. Offering two options allows them to practice decision-making in a manageable way, gradually building their belief in themselves.

Here are some frameworks for older children:

The Traffic Light Method is visual and intuitive:

Red: Stop. Pause and think before deciding. Assess risks or problems.

Yellow: Think. Consider your options and the possible outcomes.

Green: Go. Make your choice and act.

Example: Deciding whether to eat a snack before dinner. Red: Is this a good idea? Yellow: Eating now might spoil my appetite for dinner. Waiting means I'll enjoy dinner more. Green: Wait for dinner.

The STOP Model is a way to pause and reflect before acting:

Stop. Pause before acting. Take a breath.

Think about your choices. What options do you have?

Outcome consideration. What might happen for each choice?

Pick the best choice. Decide and act.

Example: Deciding whether to play video games or do homework. **S**top: Pause before acting impulsively. **T**hink: Consider the options (play games now or do homework first). **O**utcomes consideration: Playing now means staying up late to finish homework; doing homework first leaves more time to relax. **P**ick: Choose to complete homework first.

The 3Cs Model encourages children to consider consequences and take responsibility:

Choices: What options do I have?

Consequences: What will happen with each choice?

Choose: Pick the best option based on what's right.

Example: Whether to tell the truth about accidentally breaking a vase. **C**hoices: Admit it or try to hide it. **C**onsequences: Telling the truth may lead to a discussion, but lying might create more trouble later. **C**hoose: Decide to admit the mistake.

The WANT-Need Framework helps children prioritize competing demands. It assists with making more mindful, intentional decisions by considering both the short-term and long-term consequences of fulfilling desires versus meeting genuine needs.

W: What do I **w**ant?

A: What do I **A**ctually need?

N: **N**ow or later?

T: **T**hink and decide.

Example: Deciding whether to spend allowance on candy or save for a toy. **W**ant: I want candy now. **A**ctual need: I must save for the toy I've been dreaming of. **N**ow or later: Can I wait and enjoy something more significant later? **T**hink and decide: Choose to save for the toy.

Intuition

Intuition is understanding or knowing something without thinking, reasoning, or analysis. People often describe it as a "gut feeling", "good or bad vibes", or an instinctive perception. It is internal knowledge that operates beneath the surface of conscious awareness and is frequently accompanied by strong emotional signals.

Teaching your child about intuition involves helping them recognize, trust, and use their inner sense of knowing while encouraging reflection and logical analysis. Use simple language to describe intuition as their "inner voice" or a "gut feeling" that helps them decide or understand situations. Example: "Intuition is when you just have a feeling about something without knowing exactly why."

Encourage them to listen to these feelings and sensations. Teach them to pay attention to how they feel in different situations, such as meeting new people, trying new things, or making decisions. Ask them questions like, "How does this make you feel inside?" or "Does this feel right to you?"

Guide them to pay attention to physical sensations, like a sense of unease or excitement, which can guide their direction. If something doesn't feel right, it's worth pausing to figure out why. Teach them to slow down, take time to carefully consider decisions, and notice their thoughts and feelings while doing so. When the body and mind are still, it becomes easier to tune into that inner voice.

Teach them that, while intuition is helpful, it's best to balance it with logic. It's valuable to think analytically and gather information, then check it with intuition and reasoning to ensure it's the right choice. This is especially important for big decisions. If their gut feeling warns them or raises a red flag, encourage them to investigate further. Tell them it's OK to trust their instincts but use thinking skills to back it up. Using both resources will help them make well-informed and carefully considered decisions.

Summary

Developing thinking, solving, and deciding abilities means equipping your children with the tools to face a world filled with obstacles and potential.

Critical thinking helps children analyze situations and make informed decisions by posing questions and encouraging a deeper examination of issues.

Problem-solving is not just about finding the right answer, but about understanding how to think through issues logically and systematically. It prepares them for real-world situations, instilling a sense of agency.

Decision-making encourages them to make choices, even in minor matters. It builds determination, teaches them about responsibility, and lays the groundwork for more significant decisions they'll face as they mature.

Together, these skills form a framework that encourages a proactive rather than reactive approach to life's difficulties.

Make a Difference With Your Review

Would you take a moment to help someone just like you—eager to raise strong, confident kids but unsure where to begin?

My goal with *Raising Resilient Children* is to make raising empowered, adaptable kids easier for every parent, teacher, or caregiver. But I can't do it alone.

Most people pick books **based on reviews**. By sharing your thoughts, you're not just reviewing a book—you're giving someone else the tools they need to raise resilient kids.

It's free, quick, and incredibly impactful. Simply scan the QR code below to leave a review:

If you believe in helping others, thank you for being part of this mission. Your kindness means the world to me—and to the parents and children you're supporting.

With gratitude,

Lee Alexander

Chapter Six

Autonomy and Independence

Imagine your child standing in the kitchen with a determined look, attempting to make a sandwich independently for the first time. Their small hands fumble with the peanut butter jar, but they persist, their face a mix of concentration and pride. This simple act of spreading peanut butter on bread is more than just a task; it is a step towards individuality. It is a moment where they feel capable and empowered, taking control of a small but meaningful part of their world. While the sandwich might be messy or imperfect, the process itself matters most—it builds self-reliance and reinforces the belief that they can tackle challenges by themselves.

Reflection Exercise

How often do I step in to make choices for my children?

Do I give them options and let them choose?

Can they manage basic self-care tasks without help?

Do they complete their assigned tasks without constant reminders?

Do they seek advice when necessary?

How often do they plan for events or deadlines without prompting?

Do they take ownership of their actions, including mistakes?

How reliable are they in following through on commitments?

Autonomy

Autonomy is the ability to make decisions in alignment with one's values, beliefs, and interests. In childhood, autonomy is not about complete self-sufficiency, but about exercising choice and self-direction within a supportive framework. It means empowering children to engage in decision-making processes and understand the reasoning behind their actions. Encouraging autonomy helps children build confidence and learn accountability, skills that are essential for making informed decisions throughout life.

Approaches to Increase Autonomy

For **preschoolers**, the journey toward autonomy begins with small but significant steps, such as:

- Picking out clothes.
- Deciding which book to read before bedtime.
- Deciding in which order they want to complete their nighttime routine (brush teeth, bath, snack, story).
- Letting them choose a snack and serving themselves.
- Choosing their treat at the grocery store.

School-age children can manage more significant decisions, such as:

- Allowing them to plan the weekly dinner menu.
- Choosing the weekend activity.
- Personal choices like hairstyles and clothing.
- Exploring new hobbies or interests, even if they might fail initially.
- Choosing what they want for their school lunch and then selecting healthy options at the grocery store.

For **tweens**, it is appropriate to involve them in more substantial decisions, such as:

- How to arrange their room.
- What extracurricular activities to pursue.
- Arranging their schedules and managing responsibilities like homework, chores, and free time.
- Giving them an allowance and letting them decide how to save or spend it.
- Letting them pack their bags for school, sports, or trips.

- Deciding on a family holiday destination.

Try to respect their decisions and accept the outcomes, even if the result isn't ideal. This reinforces certainty in their decision-making abilities and helps them learn from their mistakes. Example: "You brought your small backpack for the trip. Next time, you might realize a bigger one would fit everything better."

Autonomy is a journey, not a destination. It requires patience, encouragement, and a willingness to let go. Allow them to make a mess and learn through trial and error. In the process, they will discover their likes and dislikes, as well as their strengths and capabilities.

Independence

Closely tied to autonomy, independence is the ability to function without relying on others for help. Empowering children to complete tasks by themselves develops their competence and self-belief. They feel empowered and capable, which contributes to a positive self-image.

Encouraging independence in children is an investment in their future success. But it involves more than just assigning tasks. It requires an environment where they can explore, fail, and try again.

Offering guidance without taking over is key. Urge them to think analytically, weigh options, and make decisions. This approach teaches them to trust their judgment and learn from their experiences. By providing a safe space for them to explore and occasionally fail, you help them build grit and fortitude.

Here are some examples and situations for age-appropriate independence:

Preschool: Put toys away, dress themselves, sweep floors, wipe counters, feed pets, water plants, set the table, wash hands.

School-age: Make simple snacks, keep their room tidy, bathing, grooming, unloading the dishwasher, folding clothes, brush the pet.

Tween: Cook simple meals, keep track of allowance, save money for a desired goal, homework, do their own laundry, care for siblings, walk the dog.

You can help by creating clear expectations for tasks and establishing daily routines. Expectations encourage accountability, and routines provide structure. Please resist the urge to do tasks for them or correct every slight mistake. This will allow them to take ownership of their actions and learn from experience.

This journey requires patience, encouragement, and trust as your children learn to spread their wings and discover their capabilities. Your role is to guide them with advice and support. By facilitating independence, you empower your children to face their troubles with adaptability and strength, ready to flourish in the dynamic world that awaits them.

Digital Identity

Children must learn how to manage their online identity safely and respectfully when they create their own email and social media accounts. A positive online reputation can open doors to future opportunities and help them build meaningful connections. Conversely, a negative online status can harm their offline relationships and significantly hinder their future prospects.

Teach them what constitutes inappropriate pictures and gestures on social media and that they should not post or share these. They may not fully realize that once something is posted, it can be difficult to remove and may be viewed by future employers, colleges, or even strangers with bad intentions. It's important to think before they post, as everything they share online reflects their character and can have long-term consequences.

Encourage your children to pause and reflect before they write anything online. Teach them to evaluate the content they "like" or "share," instilling a sense of responsibility and integrity. By developing these habits, they can avoid impulsive decisions and work on building an online identity that aligns with their values and goals.

Positive interactions and respectful communication online are also mandatory. Children should understand that inappropriate or harmful online behavior can have real-world repercussions. Remind them that kindness and respect should extend to the virtual world, the same as in face-to-face interactions. When children grasp the lasting impact of their words and actions, they are more likely to engage positively with others. By being mindful of what you share, you can make wise choices and build a positive digital footprint.

Responsibility

Teaching children responsibility is a compelling way to nurture their personal growth and character development. When children do chores, tasks, or jobs, they learn to follow through on commitments and become accountable, an experience that boosts self-efficacy. This gradual process helps them understand the value of hard work and the satisfaction of contributing to the greater good. They see themselves as capable and reliable individuals, laying the groundwork for tenacity and self-reliance.

Responsibility develops through a series of steps, each building on the last. It starts with small tasks that give children control and ownership over their environment. These tasks, however simple they seem, establish the basis for more significant duties in the future.

For **preschoolers**, responsibility begins with modest chores, like putting toys away or helping set the table. These activities teach them about contributing to the family and understanding their role within the household. As they age, you can assign them more complex tasks, like making their bed or helping with grocery lists. Each new assignment gives a sense of accomplishment and self-reliance.

As children enter **school-age**, their capacity for more complex responsibilities increases. They can assist with household chores like cleaning their room, washing dishes, or folding laundry. They may also be capable of caring for the family pet. Such activities instill a sense of pride and accomplishment, essential for building a strong work ethic and understanding the importance of perseverance.

Tweens are ready to embrace more substantial responsibilities, both personal and academic. Encourage them to take ownership of their schoolwork and manage their schedules. These practices teach them to balance various aspects of their lives, a skill crucial for adulthood. Be available as a sounding board but avoid dominating their decisions. This approach helps them develop critical thinking and problem-solving skills, reinforcing their ability to make informed choices and learn from their mistakes.

One effective way to track responsibilities is by creating a visual chart that outlines tasks for each family member. This chart can serve as both a reminder and a motivator, helping children see their contributions to the household.

As they complete tasks, encourage them to reflect on their experiences. Ask questions like, "What did you learn from this?" or "How did you feel after finishing?" These reflections help them internalize the lessons learned from their responsibilities, contributing to their overall maturation.

Risk-Taking

Often misunderstood, risk-taking has connotations of danger and recklessness. Yet, in children's development, it can be a valuable tool for betterment and learning. The adage, "Nothing ventured, nothing gained," rings true, as taking risks helps children build confidence and self-assurance.

When guided appropriately, risk-taking allows children to explore their capabilities and expand their comfort zones safely and constructively. When children step out of their "default settings," they learn to have faith in their abilities, which enhances their self-esteem and determination.

Risk-taking is pivotal in building resilience, as it involves facing failure directly. Children learn to pick themselves up after a setback, recognizing that failure is not the end, but a pathway to improvement. This mindset leads to adaptability, equipping them to handle life's unpredictable contests.

It's imperative to clarify the distinction between reckless and constructive risks. **Reckless** risks are those taken without forethought or planning, often leading to unnecessary harm. In contrast, **constructive** risks are calculated, involving a thoughtful assessment of potential outcomes. Encouraging children to take constructive risks fosters advancement, allowing them to explore new possibilities and build self-efficacy.

You play a pivotal role in guiding your children through this process:

1. First, they should assess the situation carefully: Identify any obvious dangers (e.g., slippery surfaces, sharp objects, moving vehicles). Discuss key factors that may affect the outcome (e.g., how much experience they have in the activity, whether they have the necessary skills). Understand the environment (e.g., Are there rules in place? Are adults nearby for guidance if needed?).

2. Next, you can direct them to weigh the pros and cons. Pros: What could they gain from taking this risk? (e.g., Learning a new skill, gaining confidence, having fun). Cons: What could go wrong? (e.g., Possible injuries, failure, disappointment).

3. Analyze potential outcomes together. Guide them to think through the possible consequences of their decision. What is the worst-case scenario, and how could they handle it? What is the best-case scenario, and what would they gain? What is the most likely outcome?

4. Decide and act: If the risk is reasonable and they feel ready, encourage them to go for it. If they decide against it, reinforce that choosing not to take a risk is also a valid and smart decision.

When they succeed, celebrate their achievements with them. When they stumble, offer encouragement and guidance to help them learn from the experience. This balanced approach builds self-determination and instills courage, empowering them to embrace life's uncertainties fearlessly.

At the **preschool** stage, children are learning basic physical and social skills. Non-reckless risks involve trying new things within a supervised environment, such as:

- Climbing on playground equipment.
- Jumping off a low step or small ledge under supervision.
- Riding a balance bike or tricycle.
- Introducing themselves to a new peer.
- Sharing toys and taking turns.
- Exploring new art materials like paints or clay.

Children in the **school-age** range are becoming more independent and curious, making it an excellent time for bigger challenges, including:

- Trying a new sport.
- Riding a bike without training wheels.
- Climbing a tree.
- Inviting a new classmate over for a playdate.
- Performing in front of others, such as reading a poem or singing in a school talent show.
- Joining a new club or team, like scouts or robotics.
- Reading a book without pictures.

Tweens are developing their identities and learning to take on more responsibility, making it a good time to explore activities that push their boundaries in safe ways, such as:

- Taking on a leadership role in clubs.
- Trying a new adventure activity at a supervised facility, like kayaking or rock climbing.
- Training for and completing a fun run or bike race.
- Volunteering to speak in front of the class or take part in a debate.
- Organizing a group outing or planning a small event with friends.

- Reaching out to a new peer group.
- Standing up for someone being mistreated.
- Learning a new instrument, coding skill, or complex craft like knitting.
- Taking responsibility for a long-term project, like growing a garden or raising funds for a cause.
- Exploring topics outside their comfort zone, such as public speaking or creative writing.

Encouraging non-reckless risk-taking builds children's bravery while teaching them to assess danger and manage setbacks. Supervision and support are key to ensuring these activities remain safe and beneficial.

When approached thoughtfully, risk-taking becomes a tool for empowerment. It teaches children to believe in themselves, face challenges with an open mind, and adapt to changes. They discover their strengths and weaknesses and that meaningful growth often lies just beyond their comfort zone.

Summary

Autonomy is about helping children make decisions aligned with their values while learning through choice and natural consequences within a supportive environment. As children grow, encouraging autonomy through age-appropriate decisions builds confidence, accountability, and self-awareness.

Closely linked, independence focuses on empowering children to complete tasks on their own, developing competence, resilience, and self-trust. By providing guidance without overstepping, parents foster the skills children need to navigate challenges and thrive independently in the real world.

Teaching children responsibility through age-appropriate tasks helps build their self-efficacy, work ethic, and sense of contribution. By gradually increasing responsibilities and encouraging reflection, parents foster critical thinking, perseverance, and the foundations for lifelong self-reliance.

Risk-taking encourages children to step outside their comfort zones. Through calculated risks, they explore their potential, discovering strengths they never knew they had.

Chapter Seven

Adaptability and Ingenuity

Adapting and adjusting to today's hectic world is becoming an inescapable part of modern life. These skills determine survival in the natural world and define success and achievement in human endeavors. Encouraging adaptability equips your children to explore alternative solutions and diverse approaches. Creativity encourages them to think outside the box and discover unconventional strategies. Ingenuity sparks innovation, and resourcefulness teaches children to make the most of what they have.

Perseverance is often the key ingredient that separates the successful from the unsuccessful. These qualities help children embrace change with an open heart and a flexible mind. It results in a tenacious outlook that prepares them for future difficulties.

Reflection Exercise

How do my children respond when their routines unexpectedly change?

How do they react when introduced to new environments or situations?

Do they try different approaches to problems? Or give up easily?

Do they show creativity in figuring out solutions to dilemmas?

Are they willing to try new foods, activities, or hobbies?

How do I respond when unexpected changes disrupt our family routine?

Can I adjust my parenting strategies when they are ineffective?

Am I open to adopting new techniques or ideas?

Do I explore multiple solutions to challenges?

Flexibility

In a constantly evolving world, those who can adjust their approaches and perspectives are more likely to succeed. Flexibility allows individuals to cope with unexpected changes without becoming overwhelmed. Adaptable people are less likely to experience stress when faced with uncertainty or disruption. They are also better at identifying creative and practical solutions to problems. They are willing to rethink strategies and explore alternative approaches to complex problems.

Activities to Enhance Flexibility

Promoting flexibility in children involves exposing them to activities and experiences that encourage problem-solving, emotional regulation, and creative thinking. Flexibility is at work when a family trip takes an unexpected turn due to weather, and everyone quickly shifts to indoor activities, maintaining the spirit of adventure.

Flexibility is involved when a student discovers their usual study method isn't working academically and experiment with fresh approaches to grasp a challenging concept. By nurturing flexibility, you are empowering your children to embrace change and approach challenges with a sense of curiosity and confidence.

Here are some suggestions for **all ages**:

- Simple games like "Simon Says" can introduce them to flexibility, requiring them to switch tasks or movements on command (see chapter 3).
- Try new foods, visit unfamiliar places, or learn about different cultures through books, movies, or activities.
- Switch up daily routines, like walking a different route to school or trying a new family activity.
- Encourage brainstorming sessions where they can explore alternative solutions to a single problem, teaching them that there is often more than one way to achieve a goal.
- Play an improvisation game, where thinking on their feet is mandatory.
- Present hypothetical scenarios and ask your children how they would handle them. Example: "What if it suddenly started raining during your picnic?"
- Take spontaneous trips, or plan "mystery outings" where you

- don't reveal the destination or activity until arrival.
- Play the "Yes and....." game. One person begins with a statement: "We're going on a road trip!" The next person responds, "Yes, and..." and then adds a new idea or detail.
- Share examples from your life where you had to adapt or stay flexible.
- Model how to handle unexpected changes calmly and positively.

Creativity

Creativity breathes life into problem-solving, transforming barriers into prospects for innovation. It's about thinking radically, exploring unconventional solutions, and allowing imagination to guide. When children tap into their creativity center, they unlock a world of possibilities where no idea is too wild and no solution too improbable. Creative thinking also builds confidence, teaching children that their ideas hold value and potential.

A playful approach to roadblocks often leads to the most innovative solutions. Viewing problems as puzzles to solve can transform daunting tasks into engaging adventures. When humor is used to approach difficult situations, it diffuses tension and opens the mind to new possibilities. This lighthearted attitude fosters originality as children learn to face barriers with curiosity and optimism.

Nurturing Creativity

Activities that boost creativity encourage children to experiment, take risks, and learn from failures. Here are just a few suggestions for **preschoolers**:

- Add a new layer to simple art projects by asking them to create a story to explain or accompany the artwork. This builds narrative skills alongside creativity.
- Set up sensory bins with materials like sand, water, or rice, allowing them to experiment and discover kinesthetically.
- Avoid toys with fixed outcomes (e.g., battery-operated toys with limited functions).
- Set up a dress-up corner with costumes and props.
- Role-play scenarios like running a store, cooking, or being a doctor.

- Introduce simple musical instruments like tambourines or xylophones.

School-age children might benefit from the following activities:

- Provide science kits, cooking projects, or simple coding games where they can explore and test ideas.
- Activities like making friendship bracelets, building model airplanes, or designing greeting cards allow them to personalize projects.
- Present fun challenges, like building the tallest tower with marshmallows and toothpicks.
- Let them create their own recipes or decorate cookies. Discuss how combining ingredients can result in something new.
- Encourage group projects like writing a play, building a fort, or painting a mural with friends.

Tweens, with their increasing independence, can engage in more complex projects such as:

- Photography, journaling, and songwriting. It enables them to explore their unique style.
- Coding, video editing, animation, or graphic design. Encourage them to create photo collages, YouTube videos, or digital art.
- Take them to art museums, live theater, or concerts to inspire them.
- Introduce books, documentaries, or biographies about creative individuals.

Resourcefulness

Picture yourself: a kitchen, minimal ingredients and hungry people. The pantry is sparse, yet dinner needs to be on the table soon. This scenario illustrates the real-world application of resourcefulness. It's about using what you have to solve problems creatively. Resourcefulness isn't just a skill; it's a mindset that transforms limitations into opportunities.

When children learn to think resourcefully, they develop ingenuity, effortlessly adapting to changing circumstances. This ability to find innovative solutions builds self-reliance. It teaches them to embrace difficulty rather than shy away from it.

Stimulating Resourcefulness

Encouraging children to think imaginatively and make the most of the supplies they have is at the core of resourcefulness. Below are some practical ideas to stimulate this trait in your children:

Have a brainstorming session where they list all possible uses for a common item, such as a paperclip or a rubber band. This encourages them to view everyday objects from new perspectives.

The "MacGyver" challenge: Provide a collection of random household items (e.g., toilet paper rolls, bread bag clips, empty food containers). Give them an objective, like building a bridge that can hold weight, creating a tool to pick up an object, or making a simple toy.

Build a survival kit: Pretend you're camping, stranded on an island, or facing a natural disaster. Ask your children to list essential items they would pack or use. Discuss why they chose each item and explore how they might adapt if something they needed wasn't available.

Pose scenarios such as "What if you were lost in a store? What would you do?" "How would you communicate if your phone didn't work?" Let them act out or explain their solutions.

Inspire them to start a small business, like a lemonade stand or a craft shop. They must figure out how to make their product with what's available, market it, and "sell" it to family members, friends, or neighbors.

Have them invent their own board game using basic materials (paper, markers, small objects for tokens). They must come up with rules, objectives, and a playable format. Play the game together and discuss ways to enhance it.

Set up a mini obstacle course indoors or outdoors (e.g., climb over a chair, crawl under a table). Give them "tools" like a rope or blanket to help them complete the course. Let them brainstorm different ways to use the tools creatively.

Give them a pile of toy building blocks or materials and have them create a specific object (e.g., a car, a house) without instructions. Encourage them to redesign if their first idea doesn't work.

Here are some more simple but effective ideas:

- Rearrange furniture to create more space in a room.

- Do-it-yourself craft projects from recycled materials. For example, you can turn old clothes into costumes or stuffed animals.

- Fix a broken toy using only materials found in the house.

- Christmas gift exchange using a $0 budget with items found at home.

- Let them create meals using limited ingredients. Ask them to suggest substitutions if a key ingredient is missing.

- Go camping with minimal store-bought supplies. Help them find natural items to build shelter, cook food, and provide warmth.

Perseverance

Perseverance is the determination to keep going, to try again, and to push through barriers with resolve. It's a crucial component of resilience, enabling children to develop grit and tenacity. Through perseverance, children learn failures are not the end of the road but an inevitable detour along the way. They discover the value of repeated effort and the priority shifts from immediate results to the journey of improvement and learning.

In adulthood, perseverance is often the defining factor between success and failure. It forces those driven to succeed to maintain concentration, adapt to problems, and continue striving despite difficulties. These qualities are essential for personal development, academic achievement, and long-term success in all aspects of life.

Attainment of significant and long-term endeavors requires sustained effort. Perseverance helps individuals break down larger goals into manageable steps. It's what drives them to continue building and working, even when progress is slow. Over time, this strengthens self-efficacy and self-worth.

Reflection Exercise

How do my children react to a difficult or unfamiliar task?

Have I observed them persisting through frustration?

How often do they retry a task after failing the first time?

Do they brainstorm alternative approaches?

How do I stay motivated for objectives that require sustained effort?

When faced with obstacles, do I seek solutions or feel discouraged?

Am I willing to delay gratification to attain long-term objectives?

Developing Perseverance

Start by shifting the emphasis off outcomes and onto effort and progress, as discussed in Chapter 4: Growth Mindset. The following sections detail further suggestions:

Create a "Challenge of the Week": Start a family contest that requires effort and persistence. Examples include completing a puzzle, running a specific distance, or memorizing a poem. Celebrate together when they complete the objective.

Implement the "Try Three Times" Rule. Set the expectation that your children must attempt to solve their problems at least three times before asking for help or moving on. Apply this to simple tasks, like opening a jar, tying a knot, or solving a math equation.

Discuss feelings around the topic of quitting. Help them reflect on how it feels to give up versus how it feels to succeed after trying hard. Ask questions like, "How did you feel when you finished the hard part?" or "What helped you keep going?"

Here are some other ideas to consider:

- Share stories about times you overcame obstacles.
- Verbalize your thought process: "This is tricky, but I'll keep trying until I figure it out."
- Break larger goals into smaller, more manageable steps. This approach helps children to see their progress clearly, motivating them to continue.
- Celebrate the small victories, recognizing that each step forward is a triumph.
- Play long board games that require patience.
- Introduce activities where persistence is necessary to succeed, such as gardening, knitting, learning a different language or playing an instrument.
- Read books or watch movies about famous individuals or characters who overcame struggles through determination.

Change

There is a Buddhist teaching that says, "Nothing is permanent." Indeed, the only constant in today's landscape is change. Transitions are like the shifting sands beneath children's feet, sometimes unsettling, often unpredictable. They can be as small as moving up a grade or as significant as relocating to a new city. Each transition brings unique tests and trials, potentially affecting children's well-being.

Children thrive on routine, so when familiar patterns change, it can lead to uncertainty and anxiety. This upheaval requires them to cope with new environments and adjust their sense of security. Yet, these transitions also provide occasions to teach adaptability and perseverance. When children learn to prevail over change, they develop the ability to face life's unpredictability with self-assurance.

Reflection Exercise

Do my children adapt their behavior in a dynamic environment?

How do they interact with new people?

How willing are they to try new routines or activities?

How effectively do I adapt my strategies to new circumstances?

How willing am I to embrace new ideas and perspectives?

Am I receptive to feedback?

Supporting Children Through Change

The first strategy is to **model positive behavior** yourself. Be calm and use effective coping techniques during transitions. Children imitate their parents, so if you remain composed and positive, your children are more likely to do the same.

Communication is paramount during times of change. Children generally like to know what's coming and what to expect. Providing clear, timely information about the upcoming transition allows them to prepare emotionally and mentally. Letting them know well in advance will enable them to process the information at their own pace, reducing feelings of uncertainty or anxiety.

Setting clear expectations about their role in the transition will reduce uncertainty and anxiety. It will help them approach the transition with greater peace and calm. Use age-appropriate language to explain the situation in terms they can understand. It's best to avoid overly complex or vague descriptions that might confuse or worry them.

Open dialogue creates a safe environment where children feel comfortable expressing their feelings, fears, and questions without judgment. This openness validates their emotions and helps them articulate concerns they might not fully understand or know how to process. Encouraging them to share their thoughts supports emotional expression and helps with emotional regulation amidst the uncertainty. When appropriate, involving them in discussions about the transition can empower them and make them feel included.

Let them **make decisions** about the change. This will provide a sense of control. For instance:

- If you are moving, let them choose which bedroom they want and how to decorate it.
- If they are starting a new school, let them choose between two after-school activities.
- If a new baby is coming, let them help choose names, prepare the nursery, and buy supplies.

These may seem insignificant, but it makes a world of difference for children to have some choice in a situation that may feel out of their control.

Gradual exposure to change can help children adapt more efficiently. Incremental adjustments are far more palatable for children than a sudden large shift all at once. For example, if your family is moving to a new home, you can visit the new neighborhood several times before moving. You can explore local parks, shop at nearby stores, and drive by the new house frequently. This gradual introduction allows your children to adjust at their own pace, making the change feel less overwhelming and more approachable.

Stories and play can be practical tools for helping children cope with change. Reading books that address similar situations allows children to see their feelings reflected and validated. It helps them understand their sentiments are expected and normal. Additionally, role-playing scenarios related to the change provide a safe way for children to process their thoughts and feelings. This interactive technique helps them prepare and builds confidence in the upcoming transition.

The key is listening and validating their feelings, letting them know their thoughts matter. This support builds trust and reinforces that you are their rock in changing or difficult times.

Summary

Teaching children to be adaptable and resourceful is indispensable in a world that shifts and changes with every breath. These qualities empower them to face troubles head-on and persist through them, even though it may be difficult. By cultivating these traits, you prepare them to succeed in environments that are as unpredictable as they are exciting.

Adaptability allows them to pivot gracefully when plans change, while creativity fuels their ability to find novel solutions to complex problems. Resourcefulness encourages them to make the most of what they have. Perseverance teaches them to keep moving forward, even when the path is steep and rocky.

Change is inevitable, but how one responds to it determines success and defines the journey.

Chapter Eight

Conflict

Children encounter various forms of conflict daily, each with unique variables. From playground disputes to digital disagreements, these experiences test their emotional regulation, stress tolerance, and fortitude. Unresolved conflicts can erode self-esteem, strain relationships, and create a sense of helplessness.

Conflicts can be intimidating for children, but they also present enrichment opportunities. Teaching conflict resolution skills from a young age is beneficial in preventing minor issues from escalating into more significant problems. Children gain certainty in handling future conflicts when they approach disagreements with a mindset geared toward resolution. Though stressful and sometimes upsetting, conflict presents a fantastic occasion to deepen connections, increase empathy, and generate self-efficacy.

Reflection Exercise

What types of situations cause my children the most conflict?

How well do they manage reactions to their triggers?

How do they handle situations where their needs or desires aren't met?

Do they try to find solutions to conflicts or avoid addressing the issue?

How do they react to constructive criticism or feedback?

Do I model the conflict resolution skills I wish to instill in my children?

What guidance have I given my children to manage conflict?

Resolution Strategies

Conflict resolution is an acquired skill vital for personal and social development. It's not something most people are born with or are naturally good at. For most people, it is very uncomfortable. As with other skills in this book, you must practice conflict resolution to become good at it. As a parent, modeling conflict resolution is one of the most valuable tools at your disposal.

Your actions and reactions in everyday disagreements provide a blueprint for your children. Demonstrating how to negotiate disputes constructively shows your children that conflicts are opportunities to learn from and connect more deeply with one another. This approach creates a family culture rooted in trust and respect.

One preventative strategy is to help your children identify their triggers. Assist them in determining what sets them off emotionally and encourage them to either walk away, or pause, breathe, and reflect before responding. Anger might flare, but it need not control the outcome. Encourage them to express emotions constructively in any way suggested in Chapter 3.

Once a conflict has ensued, begin with active listening and understanding the other person's perspective. Push your children to listen to others, not just with their ears, but their hearts. Validation is equally important, as conflicts tend to dramatically de-escalate when the disgruntled person feels heard and understood. This practice promotes empathy, allowing them to see beyond their viewpoint and into others' worlds.

Using "I" statements is also very helpful. It allows an individual to express feelings without casting blame. Instead of saying, "You never listen," they might say, "I'm feeling ignored." This subtle shift encourages open dialogue and reduces defensiveness.

Several purposeful strategies are outlined below for you to coach your children if their conflicts cannot be solved using any of the above approaches.

Focus on the Problem, Not the Person

This strategy aims to separate the actual issue from the individual involved. The rationale for this is to avoid personal attacks and hurt feelings. Conflicts are common, but they do not need to escalate into detrimental words directed at the core of who a person is. Permanent hurt and damage to relationships happen when people stoop to this level. Focusing on the problem is effective because it encourages collaboration instead of hostility. Example: "The issue is that we have different ideas about completing the project, not that you're wrong or I'm right."

"Win-Win"

Teaching children the "win-win" approach means guiding them to find solutions that satisfy everyone involved. In this scenario, no one is giving up a portion of what they want. This is achieved by considering everyone's needs and brainstorming solutions. For example, if two children want to play with the same ball, you might ask, "You want to play with the ball, and your friend wants to play with it too. How can you both use it?" This prompts children to think creatively and collaboratively, leading to agreeable outcomes for all parties while building problem-solving and negotiation skills.

Seek Common Ground

This resolution method identifies shared interests, values, or goals between conflicting parties. First, each party should share their perspective while the other listens without interruption. Then, take turns validating each other's feelings by paraphrasing what they've said, ensuring both feel heard and respected.

Next, ask questions to uncover common values, objectives, or desires behind the conflict. For example, "What outcome would make both of you happy?" or "What's most important to each of you in this situation?" This redirects attention from opposing positions to shared priorities, creating a sense of partnership. Frame the conversation in terms of teamwork, using inclusive language like "we" and "us" to emphasize collaboration. Example: "How can we work together to solve this problem?"

The next step is to generate ideas that meet the shared interests identified earlier. Once a list of options is made, the last step is to agree on a path forward. Include specific actions and responsibilities for each party to ensure clarity and commitment to the agreed resolution.

The SIP Method

Statement: Person A clearly states to Person B their observations or feelings about the conflict in a neutral, nonjudgmental way. They use factual language and avoid blaming or accusatory tones. This prevents defensiveness by centering on facts or personal feelings rather than assumptions.

Impression: Person A shares how the situation has affected them and the impression it has left. They use "I" statements to convey their perspective and feelings. This builds understanding by allowing Person B to see how their actions have affected Person A. It also keeps the focus on feelings rather than blaming.

Pull for perspective: Person A invites Person B to share their perspective or clarify their intentions. They ask open-ended questions to understand Person B's point of view better. This promotes empathy by allowing them to justify their actions or feelings. It also helps uncover misunderstandings and common ground. Examples of pull statements include, "But I'm wondering what was going on for you?" "Can you help me understand what you were thinking at that moment?" or "What are your goals or concerns in this situation?"

Here's an example of the SIP Method: Your child and their classmate, Sam, are working on a team project. Your child feels frustrated because Sam often submits their work late, causing delays in their portion of the project.

Statement: "Sam, I noticed that the last couple of deadlines for our project have been missed, and we've had to rush to complete things on time."

Impression: "This makes me feel stressed because I worry about the quality of our work and meeting the overall project deadline. It also feels like I carry more workload when tasks are late."

Pull for perspective: "I'd like to understand what's been going on from your side. Is there something that's been making it hard to meet the deadlines?"

Outcome: Your child and Sam discuss solutions together, such as creating a shared schedule, breaking tasks into smaller pieces, or asking for additional support from the teacher as needed.

The SIP method ensures the conversation remains constructive, converging on the issue rather than assigning blame. It encourages both parties to hear and understand each other without rushing to judgment. Inviting the other person to share their perspective shows that their thoughts and feelings are valued. Escalation is prevented by avoiding accusatory language, reducing the likelihood of defensiveness.

Compromise

This method involves finding a middle ground where all parties are satisfied. However, it usually requires one or both people to give up something. Compromise begins with respect for others' opinions, feelings, and needs. It requires acknowledging that different perspectives are valid and everyone can express their viewpoints.

Compromise requires a willingness to adjust one's stance and consider alternatives. This flexibility is essential for finding solutions that work for everyone. Effective compromise involves fairness, where no one feels coerced or that they are giving up too much. The end arrangement should make all parties feel their concerns have been considered and addressed.

Steps in the compromise process:

1. Identify the issue: Clearly define what the disagreement is about to ensure everyone is addressing the same concern.
2. Understand priorities: Each party should articulate their foremost needs or wants, distinguishing between negotiable and non-negotiable points.
3. Explore options: Brainstorm multiple solutions, encouraging creativity and collaboration.
4. Evaluate solutions: Discuss the feasibility and fairness of each option, aiming for an outcome that satisfies everyone's key priorities.
5. Agree and implement: Decide on the best course of action and ensure all parties commit to the agreed-upon solution.

Agree to Disagree

This solution recognizes that some conflicts may not have a clear resolution, and it's okay to maintain differing opinions. It is effective because it preserves relationships by stopping and moving on from the conflict. Each party must avoid personal attacks or attempts to "win" the argument. The benefit of this approach is that it maintains civility and mutual respect, even in the absence of consensus.

Example statements to conclude the interaction are below:

- "Since we're not likely to change our minds, let's respect each other's perspectives and move on."
- "While we disagree, I value how much you care about finding solutions, and we both want the best outcome."
- "I appreciate we can have open discussions, even if we don't see eye to eye."
- "We see this differently, and that's okay. Let's focus on what we can agree on."

Peer Pressure

As children mature, they look to their peers for validation. This assists them with traversing the complex social landscape of school and beyond. Peer influence can be both uplifting and detrimental.

Positive peer influences can inspire children to adopt new hobbies, strive for academic excellence, or engage in community service. However, negative influences can lead them down a path of risky behaviors, such as skipping school or experimenting with substances. Understanding this dual nature is central to guiding your children safely through these formative years.

Peer pressure plays a significant role in identity formation. During the school-age years, children explore who they are and where they fit in the world. Peer groups offer a sense of belonging, providing a mirror for children to see themselves reflected in the eyes of others. This can lead to positive growth when friendships reinforce healthy values and goals.

Yet, the pressure to conform can also stifle individuality, pushing children to suppress their true selves to fit in. Consider a nine-year-old who starts dressing inappropriately because "everyone else is doing it" or a tween who starts skipping lunch to gain acceptance from their newly formed friendship circle. This negative influence could start a cascading series of events toward more risky and harmful behavior. Over time, these small developments can erode their confidence and decision-making skills, leading to long-term issues in asserting their values and maintaining their identity.

Strategies to Address Peer Pressure

Methods to counteract peer pressure start with cultivating strong **self-esteem** and confidence. This serves as a buffer against negative influences. Self-assured children are less likely to succumb to peer pressure because they have faith in their judgment and are satisfied with who they are.

Conversations with your children about peer pressure should be as open and honest as possible. Create a safe space at home where your children feel comfortable discussing their social experiences without fear of judgment. Keeping the lines of communication open will go a long way for you, especially if your children are inching closer to becoming teenagers. The foundation you lay now will benefit your relationship with them for years.

In order to guide their decisions, help your children **define their values and beliefs.** Talk about what matters to them and why, reinforcing that they can stick to their values even when others disagree. Ask questions that prompt them to think deeply about what matters most to them.

Here are some **thoughtful questions** to ask your children when their values and beliefs are in jeopardy. These inquiries can help them reflect on the situation, clarify their values, and decide how to respond:

- "What are some things that are important to you, no matter what others say?"
- "How do you decide if something is right or wrong for you?"
- "How do you feel when you stick to your values, even if your friends disagree?"
- "What happened that made you feel your values or beliefs were being questioned?"
- "What made you uncomfortable about the situation?"
- "How did it feel when someone questioned what you believe in?"
- "What emotions came up when you considered standing up for your values?"
- "What do you think is the right thing to do in situations like this?"
- "Why is this value or belief important to you?"
- "If you could go back, would you react the same way or differently?"
- "What's the hardest part about standing up for your values?"
- "What can you do next time to stay true to yourself?"
- "What did you learn about yourself from this experience?"
- "How can this situation help you prepare for similar ones in the future?"

Encourage **positive friendships:** Help your children build relationships with peers who share their values and make healthy choices. Encourage involvement in groups or activities that attract like-minded individuals. For example, suggest joining a sports team, club, or community group to meet positive role models. Help them explore their interests and celebrate their unique qualities, reinforcing that they don't need to change who they are to be valued.

Here are some questions you can ask them when their friendships are feeling confusing:

- "Why do you think friends sometimes pressure each other?"
- "What do you notice about how people act when trying to fit in?"
- "How do you know if someone is a true friend?"
- "How can you encourage your friends to make healthy choices too?"

When faced with a dilemma, assist your children to **evaluate choices** and consider the consequences of their actions. Teach them to question the motives and actions of others rather than mindlessly following the group. Discuss scenarios where peer influence might arise and ask them:

- "Why do you think someone would pressure you to do that?"
- "What will happen if you do this?"
- "Is this what you really want?"

You can also assist them in planning for future scenarios:

- "What can you do if you feel pressured to do something you know isn't right?"
- "Who can you talk to if you're struggling with a tough situation?"
- "What are some ways you can leave a situation if you start to feel uncomfortable?"

Demonstrating **refusal skills** and assertive communication becomes necessary when peer pressure occurs. Assertiveness doesn't mean being aggressive; it's about expressing oneself clearly and respectfully. Equip your children with phrases and strategies to say "no" boldly without damaging friendships. Practice role-playing responses, such as:

- "No thanks, that's not for me."
- "I'll pass."
- "I can't; I have other plans."
- "Why are you so interested in me doing this?"
- "Why do you care what I do?"
- "If it's no big deal, why don't you do it alone?"

- "How about we play [another activity]?"
- "I'd rather [do a different activity]."
- "I said no, and I mean it."
- "Stop asking; my answer isn't going to change."
- "I don't need to explain myself."
- "My Mom/Dad/parents won't allow that."

Use media examples, like a TV show or movie, to spark dialogue about peer dynamics. Discuss characters' decisions and the consequences they face, encouraging your children to reflect on their own choices. These discussions can lead to insights about their pressures and how they might handle them.

Summary

As humans are social creatures, conflict and drama are part of the lived experience. By equipping children with conflict-resolution skills, you help them resolve disagreements and build their capacity for empathy and understanding.

When children learn to address conflicts calmly and patiently, they are more likely to handle larger future disputes with respect and integrity.

Strong self-esteem and assertive communication form the backbone of this empowerment, enabling children to resist negative influences and embrace their unique identity.

Chapter Nine

Hardship

Children face a myriad of situations that test their resilience daily. Building resolve isn't about shielding children from inevitable difficulties but empowering them to face these challenges bravely. It's about teaching them that setbacks are not failures but chances for improvement.

When children understand that fortitude involves overcoming adversity rather than avoiding it, they develop a mindset that embraces learning and personal advancement. By supporting them through their struggles, you can help them build the qualities they need to prosper in today's and tomorrow's circumstances.

Reflection Exercise

Do my children recognize when they need help and seek support?

Do they have a reliable network to turn to in challenging times?

Do they engage in healthy habits to prevent stress?

What strategies do they use to cope with pressure or anxiety?

Are they respectful to others when angry or frustrated?

Can they identify ways they've gotten stronger because of difficulties?

Stress and Anxiety

The world can be daunting for children, and each age brings its own stressors. For preschoolers, tension might stem from simple changes like a new sibling, starting preschool, or even moving to a different bedroom. They rely heavily on routine and predictability to feel safe.

As they grow into school age, academic pressures and the intricacies of social interactions surface. Peer dynamics can be complex. The desire to fit in may weigh heavily on them.

By the time they reach their tween years, these pressures compound. Academic expectations increase, and the social landscape becomes more intricate. Peer pressure often takes center stage.

These varied stressors are all interconnected. They play a significant role in shaping how children perceive and respond to the world around them.

Prevention

Helping children manage and prevent stress necessitates an approach that addresses their physical, mental, emotional, and spiritual well-being. Each component is vital in nurturing resilience and equipping children with the tools to cope with life's trials.

In the **physical** domain, promoting healthy habits such as regular activity, adequate sleep, and balanced nutrition provides a firm base for their overall health. Exercise keeps their bodies strong and releases endorphins, which help reduce stress and enhance mood. Adequate sleep ensures they are rested and better able to handle daily pressures. A nutritious diet fuels their bodies and minds for optimal functioning.

Mentally, teaching children how to identify stressors is the first step in managing them. Practicing mindfulness or relaxation techniques can assist them in regaining a sense of calm in overwhelming situations.

Emotionally, open communication and encouraging them to express their feelings in safe and supportive environments helps them develop emotional regulation and self-awareness (see Chapter 3). Listening to their concerns without judgment validates their experiences and builds trust.

On a **spiritual** level, providing opportunities for reflection, gratitude, and connection to something greater—whether through nature, faith, or acts of kindness—can offer children a sense of purpose and grounding. Integrating these elements into their daily routines prevents stress from accumulating and equips children with lifelong skills to maintain balance and peace in the face of adversity.

Management

Coping strategies are essential in helping children manage stress and anxiety. Here is a sampling of stress prevention and reduction activities tailored to each age group. Keep trying various strategies until you find some that work for your children. Please revisit the suggestions in

Chapter 3: Techniques to Manage Emotional Outbursts. The strategies discussed there are just as effective for short and long-term stress management.

Preschoolers thrive on routine, play, and emotional connection. Stress prevention activities for this age focus on creating a sense of security and helping them express emotions:

- Use visual schedules to help them understand what comes next.
- Bring calming toys, like stress balls or weighted plushies, into the house.
- Blow bubbles to encourage slow, deep breathing.
- Take outdoor walks or play in the park to release energy and connect with nature. Encourage them to observe and name things they see, hear, or smell.
- Use simple guided imagery to help them imagine a peaceful place, like a beach or a garden. Narrate the imagery in a calm voice to help them relax.
- Introduce basic yoga poses such as cat-cow, downward dog, mountain and child's pose. Use storytelling to make yoga fun, like pretending to be animals.

School-age children benefit from activities that develop emotional awareness, problem-solving, and coping skills:

- Encourage sports, biking, or playing tag to burn off stress.
- Introduce more challenging yoga poses like tree pose, bridge, butterfly, sphinx, and plow.
- Provide a journal to write or draw about their day and feelings. Use prompts like "What made you happy today?" or "What was hard today?"
- Teach a simple body scan: Lie or sit still and concentrate on each part of the body in turn to notice how it feels. Observe objectively, without judgement and without trying to change it.
- Practice gratitude by sharing three things they're thankful for each day.
- Provide materials for DIY crafts, like making friendship bracelets or painting.
- Engage in collaborative projects like creating a family scrapbook.

- Gardening.

Tweens are facing more social, academic, and emotional predicaments. Activities should emphasize self-care, peer relationships, and personal empowerment:

- Encourage participation in sports teams or individual activities, like running or swimming.

- Introduce martial arts or dance classes for physical and mental discipline.

- Encourage hobbies like drawing, writing stories, or playing musical instruments.

- Support involvement in drama or creative writing clubs.

- Host small group hangouts with friends to build supportive relationships.

- Teach how to prioritize tasks and use planners or apps to manage homework and activities.

- Encourage involvement in community service to create a sense of purpose. Suggest simple acts like helping at a local food bank or organizing a neighborhood cleanup.

- Plan hikes, camping trips, or beach days to disconnect from technology. Teach outdoor skills like map reading or identifying plants and animals.

While many children can manage stress with the proper home support, sometimes **professional help** becomes necessary. Early intervention can make a significant difference, providing your children with the tools they need to cope. Remember, seeking help is a sign of strength, not weakness. It's about equipping your children with the resources to be healthy and happy.

Bullying

Knowing your child is a victim of bullying can leave you feeling helpless, overly defensive, and protective. It is a challenging situation that requires your immediate attention. Collaboration with the children's school or other organizations where it is occurring is also indicated.

Some of the signs of bullying may overlap with different issues or normal transient behavior in youth, so staying tuned into your children's experience is important. Maintain open lines of communication. They should feel comfortable talking to you about their day, including any troubles or concerns. Regular discussions can help you detect early signs of bullying and address them promptly.

Children who are bullied may show sudden changes in behavior or mood, such as becoming withdrawn or irritable. They might express reluctance to attend school or social events, citing vague ailments as reasons to stay home. You might notice unexplained injuries, lost belongings, or a drop in academic performance. These signs suggest your children may be facing more than just a typical schoolyard squabble.

Management of Active Bullying

Validate their experience. Listen to them without judgment or interruption. Show understanding and let them know that being bullied is not their fault. Reinforce that they were right to tell you and that you're there to support them.

Keep a detailed record of the bullying incidents. Elements to note include dates, times, locations, the people involved, what was said, who was notified, and whether any measures were taken to address the issue. This documentation will be helpful when discussing the issue with school authorities.

Contact the school or authorities. Work with teachers, counselors, and administrators to address the bullying. Share your documentation and advocate for clear actions, such as increased supervision, intervention, or mediation. Request a copy of and understand their anti-bullying policies and programs.

Regularly **meet with school officials** to discuss your children's experiences and progress. If the bullying persists or the school is unresponsive, escalate the issue to district administrators or authorities. In severe cases, particularly if threats or physical harm are involved, you may involve law enforcement.

You may also consider **temporarily pulling your children out of school** until the situation gets better, especially if the bullying threatens their safety. While this may seem like an extreme measure, bullying can sometimes escalate to severe harm, including bodily injury, psychological trauma, or even self-harm. Ensuring your child's safety and emotional well-being is the top priority. Missing school for a short period is a minor inconvenience in comparison to any of the above mentioned adverse outcomes.

Exploring **alternative educational settings**, such as transferring to a different school, may help your children have a fresh start in a more supportive and respectful environment. Many areas now offer online schooling options, providing a safe and flexible learning environment.

These proactive steps can prevent further harm and help them regain confidence, focus, and peace of mind.

Seek professional support when necessary. If the bullying has caused emotional distress, consider seeking help from a counselor or therapist. Professional guidance can help children process their feelings, rebuild their self-esteem, and develop healthy coping strategies.

Help your children practice **safe ways to respond to bullying:**

Stay calm and firm: Bullies often target individuals who react emotionally. Maintaining composure might discourage their behavior. Help them display a neutral facial expression and steady voice. Teach them to avoid showing anger, fear, or tears in the moment.

Use assertive communication: Assertiveness shows that the bullying won't be tolerated while avoiding aggression, which can escalate the situation. Use "I" statements, such as "I don't like it when you talk to me like that. Stop." Keep responses brief and direct: "Leave me alone."

Avoid engaging: Ignoring or walking away can show the bully that their behavior isn't effective, reducing their incentive to continue. Do not react to verbal taunts or provocations. Leave the situation calmly if it's safe to do so.

Stick with friends and allies: Bullies are less likely to target individuals in a group. Spend time with friends or supportive peers who can collaborate and advocate for others collectively.

Use humor to deflect: A well-placed joke or lighthearted response can disarm the bully and de-escalate the situation, such as, "Wow, you must've really practiced that insult!"

Avoid isolation: Feeling or being alone can make bullying more impactful. Building a support network helps combat its effects. Encourage them to spend time with friends and family who make them feel valued. Most importantly, reinforce to them they deserve to feel safe and respected at school and in the community.

Cyberbullying

The schoolyard has expanded into a virtual space, and with it, bullying has taken on a new form. Cyberbullying uses technology to harass, embarrass, or exclude individuals. It can be particularly harmful because it can occur 24 hours a day and reach a broad audience quickly. It also invades the home that is supposed to be children's safe space. Cyberbullying can lead to severe emotional distress, leaving children feeling isolated and powerless.

When cyberbullying occurs, you need to have a plan for how to handle it. Management of cyberbullying includes all the strategies of traditional bullying, plus these:

- Gather evidence: Save screenshots, messages, emails, or posts showing the bullying and on which platforms the incidents occurred. These records can be valuable if the situation escalates and needs to be reported.

- Teach your children how to block and report perpetrators. This can stop further harassment and signal to platforms that abusive behavior is occurring. Most social media sites have reporting tools for harassment or abuse.

Disconnecting from Social Media

Taking a break from social media can be an effective strategy to protect your children from the emotional and mental harm caused by cyberbullying. A break allows them to concentrate on their well-being without the constant pressure or anxiety of online interactions. During the break, they can engage in offline activities, strengthen real-life relationships, and rebuild self-esteem. They might resist the idea, fearing it will worsen the situation. In response, you can emphasize that it is not a punishment. It is a temporary break meant to help them feel safer.

Set a specific break period, such as a week or two, and reevaluate the decision together. In the meantime, the bullies may target your children through other means. These include text messages, emails, or in-person. They may also create fake accounts if you have blocked their primary account. Maintain open communication with your children and monitor these other channels.

Observe how your children react to being offline. Disconnecting may lead to feelings of exclusion if social media is their primary means of connecting with friends. Address this by helping them strengthen face-to-face friendships.

After the break, help your children re-enter social media gradually. Review privacy settings, remind them how to block and report users, and consider setting daily time limits to reduce overexposure. You may also consider a parental monitoring app or service to keep a closer eye on their online interactions.

Disappointment and Loss

Loss and disappointment are inevitable parts of life. While painful, these experiences shape character, build strength, and increase fortitude.

Bouncing back from disappointment also teaches children about perseverance and adaptation, valuable skills for their future. Learning to cope with loss and disappointment equips children with the resilience to press on amidst heartache. With healthy grief processing, they will eventually regain their faith in themselves and their future.

Grief is the internal experience of loss that encompasses emotional, psychological, and social dimensions. It can result from various types of loss, not limited to death. A break-up, missed opportunity, or theft of a treasured item can also spark a grief reaction. Grief also occurs in response to a symbolic loss, such as losing a cherished dream or goal.

Everyone grieves differently, and there is no "right" way to experience it. It does not need to be recognized by others to feel real to the individual experiencing it. Grief also has physical and cognitive effects, manifesting in symptoms such as fatigue, sleep disturbances, digestive ailments, difficulty concentrating, or intrusive thoughts.

Mourning is the outward expression of grief. It is influenced by cultural, social, and religious factors. It is only through mourning that grief can be resolved. Mourning rituals such as memorial services, wakes, planting a tree, or lighting candles structure the grieving process and provide occasions for social support.

Grief often comes in waves, with intense emotions periodically increasing and decreasing as time passes. Reminders of the loss can trigger these waves, like anniversaries or familiar places. Over time, the intensity of these moments usually lessens, but they may never entirely go away. Grief isn't a linear process; it's a personal journey with ups and downs. Understanding this can help your children be more patient and kinder to themselves as they heal.

Coping Strategies

Helping children process these emotions starts with validation. They are working through accepting the reality of the loss. Be present with them in their discomfort and acknowledge their feelings. This doesn't mean rushing in to fix everything and trying to make the hurt go away. It means creating a safe space for them to express themselves. Encourage them to talk about their feelings, reassuring them that sadness or anger is okay.

For preschoolers, it's important to keep explanations simple and concrete, using clear language to help them understand what has happened. Acknowledge their feelings by naming emotions, such as saying, "I see you're feeling sad." Reassure them of their safety and that it's okay to feel upset.

Storytelling and books can help them make sense of their feelings. Play-based activities using dolls or puppets provide a safe way for them to express emotions indirectly. Offer creative outlets like drawing and painting. For this age group, it is imperative to maintain consistent routines that will provide them with comfort and stability during uncertain times. Offer plenty of physical affection to soothe their worries.

For school-age children, open conversations and emotional vocabulary are key. Encourage them to share their thoughts and ask questions. It will help them articulate feelings beyond "sad" or "mad."

Normalize disappointment by explaining that it's a natural part of life. Share examples from your life if applicable. Journaling can be a helpful outlet for expressing emotions. Offer realistic optimism, such as explaining that, while it's difficult now, things will improve. Reinforce that they should be patient with themselves as they process the situation in stages.

Tweens who may experience more complex emotions like anger, guilt, or betrayal need their feelings validated without judgment. Be honest but sensitive in your explanations, as they can handle more in-depth discussions. Encourage them to explore coping strategies independently while offering support as needed.

Creative outlets like writing stories, poems, or songs about their experiences can help them process emotions. Social support is also vital—encourage them to talk to dependable friends, family, or counselors. Physical activities like sports or hiking provide a healthy way to reduce stress and boost mood. Getting involved in community service or peer support groups can help them connect with others who have faced similar situations. Be patient if they withdraw, and remind them you're always available to listen.

Rituals can play a significant role in helping children cope with loss. Creating memory books or time capsules allows them to honor their memories and celebrate what was meaningful. These activities can be therapeutic, providing closure and a tangible way to remember.

Establishing family traditions to honor loss, such as lighting a candle on anniversaries or planting a tree, can offer comfort and continuity. These rituals help children understand that while loss is a part of life, it doesn't erase the love and joy that came before. They learn that while some doors close, others offer new paths and possibilities.

Practicing gratitude can also be a therapeutic tool. Encourage your children to find silver linings, even in difficult situations. This practice helps them shift their attention from what's lost to what's still present and valuable.

Setting realistic expectations for future endeavors can also ease the sting of disappointment. It will help your children approach goals with a balanced perspective.

Support them in **finding meaning** in their loss by discussing what they learned or how they've grown from the experience. This can transform their grief into a tool for personal development, building character.

Setback and Failure

Overcoming setbacks and failure is about recognizing them as opportunities for betterment, rather than reasons to give up. Teaching children that failure doesn't define them but rather refines their path to success helps them view mistakes as stepping stones rather than roadblocks. By embracing failure as a natural part of learning, children build the determination to overcome more significant problems in the future.

When your children are actively feeling the sting of failure, the following approaches can help them process the hardship and move toward a resolution.

Address the positive first. Help them identify the aspects of the experience that went well, even if the overall outcome wasn't as expected. You might ask them, "What are you proud of in this situation?" or "What did you try that worked?" Starting on a positive note helps build their confidence and openness to learn.

Praise their effort rather than just the outcome. "I'm really proud of how hard you worked on this, even though it didn't go as planned." "Trying your best and learning from this shows how strong you are."

Encourage ownership. Teach them to take responsibility for their actions without being overly self-critical. You can ask them, "What part of this was within your control?" and "What would you do differently next time?" This approach supports them in taking accountability while avoiding blame.

Bounce Back Plan

This proactive strategy helps children recover from setbacks or failures. It provides a structured approach for regaining confidence, developing new skills, and achieving goals despite difficulties. The steps are outlined below.

1. **Acknowledge and process:** Support their emotional response. Validate their feelings, acknowledging their disappointment

without minimizing their experience. Let them express their frustrations. Reassure them it's okay to feel upset. If you allow them to truly feel their emotions, they will process them more quickly instead of getting stuck in them. Emphasize the importance of treating themselves with compassion.

2. **Analyze the situation:** Understanding what went wrong helps them to learn from the experience and avoid repeating mistakes. Identify any contributing factors: Was it a lack of preparation, external circumstances, or unrealistic goals? Ask them reflective questions like, "What could you have done differently?" Focus on what is within their control.

3. **Set realistic goals for next time:** This creates a roadmap for moving forward and regaining momentum. Break down long-term goals into smaller, achievable steps. Use SMART goals (Specific, Measurable, Achievable, Relevant, Time-Bound) to ensure clarity.

4. **Spotlight their strengths and resources:** This will boost their spirit and highlight tools for recovery. Help them identify personal strengths, such as problem-solving, creativity, or perseverance. Leverage resources like time management tools, educational materials, or supportive peers.

5. **Cultivate a positive mindset:** Maintaining optimism and centering on improvement helps sustain motivation and perseverance. Use affirmations or gratitude practices to build positivity. Emphasize progress rather than perfection.

6. **Take action:** This is the most crucial step in recovering. Begin with small, manageable steps. Monitor progress regularly and adjust plans as needed. Celebrate milestones to maintain momentum and enthusiasm.

7. **Evaluate and adjust:** Continuous reflection and adjustment ensures that the plan remains effective. Periodically review their goals, strategies, and progress. Make changes if the current methods are not yielding the desired results.

Giving Constructive Feedback

Giving constructive feedback to children is an indispensable component of rebuilding. It tempers their mood and helps them learn from their experiences. The emphasis should be on refinement rather than criticism. The feedback should be clear, specific, and solution-oriented while maintaining a positive and respectful tone. Follow these steps for the best outcome:

- **Start with positives:** Highlight what they did well. This will create a supportive atmosphere, build trust, and make them more receptive to suggestions.

- **Be specific and objective:** Avoid sounding judgmental by concentrating on specific behaviors or actions, not personality traits.

- **Use "I" statements:** Frame your feedback as your perspective to avoid sounding accusatory. "I" statements reduce defensiveness and encourage open dialogue.

- **Make suggestions:** Shift the attention from the problem to the solution. Give them practical and tangible ideas. This will motivate them to take steps toward improvement.

- **Invite dialogue:** Ask about their thoughts and encourage discussion. It will make the feedback feel collaborative rather than one-sided. Example: "What do you think? Does this suggestion feel doable for you?"

- **End on a positive note:** Reinforce your belief in their ability to advance and succeed. This will boost their self-esteem and fuel their motivation to try again.

Example: Your child didn't do well on a school project because they rushed through it. Parent: "Hey, sweetheart, can we discuss your school project? First, I want to say I'm proud of the effort you put into getting it done. You came up with some creative ideas, and I can see you worked hard on parts of it." Child: "Thanks, but I know it didn't turn out great."

Parent: "I understand you feel that way, and that's okay. Let's think about why it didn't turn out the way you wanted. I noticed you waited until the last minute to work on it. That made it hard to do your best work. What do you think?" Child: "Yeah, I guess I should have started earlier."

Parent: "I think that's a good insight! How about next time we make a plan together so you can spread the work out over a few days? That way, you'll have more time to make it great and feel proud of it. Does that sound good?" Child: "Yeah, I think that would help."

Parent: "Great! And remember, you're always learning and improving, and I'll always be here to help if you need me. I'm excited to see what you can do next time!"

Reflection

Reflection is a beneficial tool in your children's journey toward resilience. It involves looking back at experiences, analyzing them, and learning from successes and mistakes. This process develops self-awareness and helps children internalize lessons that textbooks cannot teach.

There are many ways to incorporate reflective learning into your family culture, so it will come more naturally when failures occur. One of the simplest ways is to ask open-ended questions. It helps children connect actions with outcomes. Make it routine to ask them questions such as:

- "What were you trying to achieve?"
- "What do you think you did well?"
- "What's one thing you'd do differently next time?"
- "What can this experience teach you?"
- "How will this help you next time you try something similar?"

Another simple yet effective method is creating a **"reflection jar."** Each week, children write a thought or experience on a slip of paper and drop it into the jar. At the end of the month, they can review these notes, discussing what they've learned and how they've improved. This encourages self-reflection and creates a tangible record of personal progression.

Reflection charts are a simple and effective tool for helping children think critically about their experiences. These charts can include columns with prompts such as "What happened?" "How did I feel?" and "What did I learn?" to guide their thought process. By filling out these charts, children can break down their experiences, identify emotions, and extract meaningful lessons. This structured approach makes reflection more accessible and encourages them to set the bar higher for similar situations in the future.

You may also find it beneficial to **revisit the experience** after some time has passed. It will become clear how they've grown. "Remember when you struggled with this? Look how far you've come now!" "That experience helped you become better at handling tough situations." This helps your children see their current status from a different perspective.

Signs of Distress

Signs of difficulty coping can vary from child to child. Symptoms may range from withdrawal and mood swings to changes in sleeping or eating habits. By staying attuned to these cues, you can intervene early. If your children persistently display any of these signs or their behaviors escalate, it may be time to consult a physician, school counselor, or mental health professional. Here are some of the more common signs:

- Persistent sadness, hopelessness, or frequent tearfulness.
- Excessive worry, anxiety, or fear that interferes with daily activities.
- Irritability, anger outbursts, or unusual mood swings.
- Withdrawal from friends, family, or activities they previously enjoyed.
- Difficulty concentrating, reduced academic performance, or loss of interest in school.
- Increased clinginess or dependency on caregivers.
- Risk-taking behaviors or frequent rule-breaking.
- Frequent headaches, stomachaches, or other unexplained physical complaints.
- Changes in sleeping patterns, such as insomnia or oversleeping.
- Significant changes in appetite or weight.
- Avoidance of social interactions or a sudden shift in social behavior.
- Difficulty maintaining friendships or conflicts with peers.
- Expressing thoughts of self-harm or harming others.
- Engaging in self-injurious behaviors like cutting or hitting themselves.
- Talking about feeling worthless or hopeless or wishing they hadn't been born.

Summary

Hardship touches all children and every family in some way. These experiences, while overwhelming, offer chances to teach valuable life skills. Through these trials, children develop the ability to rebound and grow stronger with each obstacle they overcome.

Creating an environment where children feel supported and understood teaches them they are not alone in their struggles. This doesn't mean shielding them from pain, but teaching them how to face it with courage and determination.

Chapter Ten

Parental Resilience

Parenting is one of life's most rewarding yet demanding roles. It requires an extraordinary balance of emotional, physical, and mental energy. However, the stresses of daily life—from work pressures, financial concerns, or the difficulties of raising a family—can weigh heavily.

Without proper attention to your needs, you risk stress, diminished patience, damage to your relationship with your children, and burnout. Taking time for self-care is important because it enables you to show up as your best self for your children.

Self-care allows you to recharge, maintain emotional balance, and build resilience. You will respond to challenges with more energy and optimism. By prioritizing your well-being, you set a positive example for your children. You are teaching them that self-care is a fundamental part of a healthy, balanced life.

Investing in self-care is not selfish; it's vital in fostering a loving, supportive environment where you and your children can thrive. In nurturing yourself, you model the very qualities you wish to instill in your children.

Reflection Exercise

What are my top three sources of stress right now?

How often do I feel overwhelmed by my responsibilities?

What specific strategies do I employ to manage stress and adversity?

What techniques do I use to stay calm and composed when angry?

Do I have enough time for myself, my family, and other responsibilities?

Am I setting realistic expectations for myself as a parent?

How much do societal or external pressures influence how I see myself?

What triggers feelings of guilt for me as a parent?

Do I compare myself to other parents, and how does this impact me?

What are my self-care strategies? Do I employ them regularly?

Stress

Parental stress can profoundly influence your children's well-being and resilience. Children are highly perceptive, often picking up on your moods and behaviors, even when not directly expressed. Feeling the weight of stress—from work pressures, financial concerns, or daily obligations—can create a ripple effect within the home. This transference of tension may lead children to mimic anxious behaviors or internalize the strain they sense. It may cause them to be unsure about expressing their emotions.

Stress doesn't simply dissipate unnoticed; it permeates the atmosphere and becomes a silent teacher. Your children learn how to approach life's difficulties through your actions and reactions. An anxious environment can inadvertently teach them to respond to adversity with fear or avoidance.

Conversely, actively managing your stress can create a calm, supportive home where peace, love, and strength abound. When you are under less stress, the entire household feels better.

Solutions

It's easy to fall into the trap of overloading yourself with tasks and commitments. Sadly, this is often driven by a fear of disappointing others, being judged, or feeling like saying "no" isn't an option. This mindset can lead to chronic overwhelm and a cycle of pressure that diminishes both your effectiveness and enjoyment of life.

What follows are some unconventional suggestions that may not be popular with your friends, relatives, or community. However, if bravely chosen, it will profoundly improve your personal and family life. You need to ask yourself, "What does happiness look like to me, and what am I willing to do to achieve it?"

Reducing your commitments is not about evading responsibilities. It is about making a conscious and deliberate choice to prioritize what truly matters most. Your time and energy are finite resources. Using them wisely is a form of self-respect. You can create a more meaningful and fulfilling life by choosing what aligns with your values and goals and discarding the rest. Letting go of unnecessary obligations opens space for deeper connections and personal growth.

Learning to say "no" is a potent tool. It allows you to preserve your mental and emotional energy for the things that align with your family's priorities and your capacity. There's not enough of you to scatter your efforts across many obligations. Saying "no" isn't a rejection of others; it's an affirmation of your boundaries and ensures that the commitments you do accept are manageable.

Simplifying your schedule helps reduce overwhelm and creates space for moments that genuinely enrich your life. With fewer competing demands, you can be more present in your interactions, especially with your children. Instead of feeling distracted or rushed, you can offer them your undivided attention, building stronger relationships and creating lasting memories. A less cluttered schedule doesn't just free up time; it brings clarity, peace, and a renewed sense of purpose to how you live and connect with those you care about.

Boundaries around your time and energy should be part of your stress management plan. This structure will increase productivity and lead to a more balanced lifestyle. Boundaries act as guardrails that protect your well-being. They ensure that each area of your life—work, family, and personal time—receives the attention it deserves without causing overload. When you intentionally define these limits, you create a sense of structure and control, reducing the chaos that often comes from an unregulated schedule.

One effective way to establish boundaries is by designating specific times for various activities. For instance:

- Implementing a "no work after dinner" rule can help you transition from professional responsibilities to quality time with loved ones. It will signal your mind and body that it's time to slow down and unwind.

- Carving out blocks of uninterrupted family time—such as a weekly game night or tech-free Sunday mornings—strengthens relationships and ensures meaningful connections.

- Personal relaxation periods, such as a daily morning walk or evening meditation, further replenish your mental and emotional reserves. You will have more stamina to meet life's demands.

These boundaries do more than organize your schedule. They create a protective buffer against the constant pull of obligations that can otherwise spill into every moment of your day. By establishing limits, you reduce the risk of burnout, enhance your focus, and prioritize what truly matters. Ultimately, this intentional approach empowers you to live with greater clarity and purpose. It allows you to recharge and bring your best self to each aspect of your life. Boundaries are not about restriction but about creating the freedom to live more fully and intentionally.

You'll likely notice a shift in your household's emotional atmosphere as you implement these strategies. You and your children can better approach life's obstacles with reduced tension, contributing to a supportive, harmonious family dynamic. This positive change can espouse deeper bonds and create a sense of stability that benefits everyone in the household.

Time Management

The demands of daily life often leave you feeling stretched thin, juggling work, family, and personal time. When schedules are packed, family connections can suffer, and meaningful interactions may take a backseat. Rushing from meetings to school pickups to household chores can make it harder to aim for building resilience. However, quality time together remains essential. Simple moments, like sharing a meal or working on a puzzle, help build trust, enrich communication, and strengthen the sense of belonging.

Solutions

Using a **family organizing app** can transform how your family circle stays connected and organized, offering a range of practical and relational benefits. One of the most significant advantages is greater coordination. With everyone's schedules, commitments, and reminders merged in one place, avoiding overlaps or forgotten responsibilities becomes easier. Features like shared calendars, task lists, and event reminders ensure everyone agrees, streamlining daily life and reducing miscommunications.

These apps also increase communication among family members. Even with varying schedules, family members can stay connected by providing a central hub for updates, messages, and shared photos or notes. This is especially helpful for larger families or those with teenagers, who might otherwise find it challenging to keep track of everyone's activities and priorities.

Another benefit of these apps is that they teach children valuable organizational skills. By involving them in planning and using the app, they learn how to manage their schedules, set reminders, and collaborate on tasks. This helps them become more responsible and prepares them for the independence required later in life.

Such apps offer features like grocery lists, meal planning, or budgeting tools, making household management more efficient. Real-time delegation and tracking of tasks and responsibilities reduces the mental load of keeping track of everything.

Hiring a housekeeper offers many practical and emotional benefits, making it a worthy investment for a more balanced lifestyle. One of the most significant advantages is the time saved by delegating routine cleaning and household chores. This allows you to zero in on work, family, or personal interests, freeing up hours to spend on things that truly matter to you. A housekeeper helps reduce stress by alleviating the burden of maintaining a tidy and organized home. The result is a calm and inviting space that you can relax in.

Beyond the practical benefits, hiring a housekeeper offers peace of mind. A consistently maintained home lets you relax and enjoy your space without worrying about pending chores. A clean and orderly environment is conducive to a more positive mindset, making your home a true sanctuary where you can unwind and recharge.

Meal delivery service subscriptions offer a range of benefits that can significantly enhance convenience, health, and quality of life. One of the primary advantages is the time saved in meal planning, grocery shopping, and preparation. For those who enjoy cooking but lack the time to shop, ingredient-based services provide everything needed for creative meal preparation while eliminating guesswork. You can also have fully prepared meals delivered to your doorstep. With these services, you can enjoy delicious, home-cooked dishes without the hassle of traditional meal preparation.

Another key benefit is the chance to discover new flavors and recipes without the effort of searching for them yourself. Many meal delivery services work with professional chefs to create diverse, restaurant-quality dishes that excite your dining routine. This allows you to explore a variety of cuisines and ingredients you might not have considered before.

Finally, subscribing to a meal delivery service can reduce stress and promote a healthier lifestyle. The knowledge that your meals are taken care of lets you focus on other priorities. Whether you're looking to save time, eat better, or explore new culinary experiences, a meal delivery service is a convenient solution that supports a busy modern lifestyle.

Limiting the number of extracurricular activities your children take part in can bring many benefits for them and you. This significantly reduces stress for your children. Overloading children with too many commitments can lead to feelings of overwhelm, leaving little time for rest, relaxation, or unstructured play. Scaling back allows them to enjoy a more balanced schedule, improving physical and emotional well-being.

Fewer activities also create more opportunities for quality family time. Families have more time to connect through shared meals, conversations, and relaxed bonding moments when a packed itinerary doesn't consume evenings and weekends. This unstructured time is essential for building stronger family relationships and creating lasting memories.

Scaling back on extracurriculars can help children explore the activities they truly enjoy and are passionate about. Rather than being stretched thin across multiple commitments, they can dedicate their energy to excelling in one or two chosen pursuits. This focus enhances skill development and teaches the value of dedication and perseverance.

Fewer activities can also ease the financial burden on family resources. Extracurricular activities often come with significant fees, equipment, or travel costs. By cutting back, you can allocate resources more thoughtfully, perhaps toward experiences that benefit the whole family or long-term goals.

Limiting extracurricular activities can lead to a more harmonious and less chaotic family dynamic. It encourages children to explore their interests without unnecessary pressure. It ensures they have time to be kids, and allows your family to maintain a healthier pace of life.

Incorporating these strategies requires intentionality, but the rewards are significant. They nurture an environment where children feel secure and supported, learning the nuances of managing time and relationships effectively. This process teaches valuable lessons in balance and prioritization, equipping your family with the tools needed to thrive.

Perceived Inadequacy

In the quiet moments after the children are finally asleep, you are haunted by thoughts of what you didn't accomplish in the day. A meeting ran late, and you missed your children's soccer game. Or perhaps you couldn't afford the latest gadget that all their friends seem to have. These are the moments when guilt creeps in.

It's a feeling as familiar as it is unjustified, stemming from the unrealistic expectations you set for yourself. Society bombards you with images of perfect parenting, leaving you to feel inadequate when you inevitably fall short of these glossy ideals. These standards are often unattainable and don't reflect the true essence of parenting.

Comparing oneself to others, especially in parenting, can be harmful and unproductive, leading to unnecessary stress, feelings of inadequacy, and strained relationships. In today's world, fueled by social media and societal expectations, it's easy to compare yourself to others who appear to "have it all together." However, these comparisons are often based on incomplete or idealized versions of reality. They create an unrealistic standard that leaves us feeling like we're falling short.

When you compare yourself to others, you risk undervaluing your unique strengths and parenting style. Every family is unique, with distinct needs, dynamics, and struggles. What works for one family may not work for another. Striving to replicate someone else's approach can lead to frustration and disconnection from your values and instincts. Comparison can breed guilt and self-doubt, distracting you from appreciating your progress and the meaningful moments you share with your children.

Comparison culture affects self-esteem and sets a damaging precedent for your children. When they observe you measuring your worth against others, they may internalize these habits and begin comparing themselves to peers. This will lead to similar cycles of insecurity. Instead of fixating on unrealistic benchmarks, it's more beneficial to celebrate your unique journey, embracing both the successes and the lessons along the way.

By letting go of comparison, you create space for gratitude and self-compassion. It will allow you to be more present and engaged with your children. Parenting isn't about perfection but connection, love, and fulfillment. By deciding on what's right for your family, you create a healthier environment for yourself and model self-acceptance for your children.

Guilt

Guilt is a common and deeply felt experience among today's parents. It arises when you believe you are falling short of the expectations you set for yourself or perceive from others. It often stems from a desire to provide the best possible upbringing for your children, coupled with the pressures of balancing multiple roles and responsibilities. Whether missing a school event due to work, losing patience in a challenging moment, or feeling you're not doing enough, you can carry a heavy emotional burden that affects your mental and emotional well-being.

Parental guilt can also manifest in different ways, depending on circumstances. For working parents, it might center on the time spent away from their children. For stay-at-home parents, it could be because they feel they aren't making enough financial contributions. Regardless of the specific trigger, the underlying theme is often a feeling of not meeting perceived expectations or letting your children down.

While some guilt can be constructive, chronic or excessive guilt can be damaging. It can lead to depression, anxiety, and a diminished sense of self-worth. It may affect the parent-child relationship. Children benefit most from parents who are present, emotionally available, and confident in their parenting. They do not benefit from parents who are consumed by guilt.

Addressing parental guilt requires a shift in perspective. **Perfection is neither attainable nor necessary**. Love, effort, and presence matter far more than meeting unrealistic standards. Practicing self-compassion involves acknowledging that parenting is a demanding journey and that facing hardship or making mistakes is natural. It means treating yourself with the same kindness, understanding, and patience that you would offer a close friend. Instead of dwelling on perceived shortcomings, remind yourself that you are doing the best you can with the resources and knowledge you have. Accept that you don't need to have all the answers or be flawless to be a great parent.

Lowering your standards and expectations can also alleviate guilt and create a more sustainable approach to parenting. This doesn't mean reducing the quality of care or love you provide, but reevaluating what needs to be done and letting go of unnecessary pressures. Relinquishing the need for a spotless house, elaborate meals, or saying yes to every obligation frees up time and energy for what truly matters: being emotionally available and present with your children. When you embrace imperfection, you model self-love and self-acceptance for your children, teaching them that being human is okay.

Focusing on your strengths and successes can help shift the narrative from guilt to empowerment. Take a moment each day to reflect on your achievements as a parent. Perhaps you managed to soothe a tantrum or made time for a meaningful conversation despite a busy schedule. These are the victories that define your parenting journey. They remind you of your capacity to nurture and support, even amidst chaos. Celebrating these moments reinforces your sense of capability, modeling a positive mindset for your children.

Connecting with other parents can also provide reassurance and support. Sharing experiences in parenting forums or groups lets you see you are not alone in your struggles. Here, stories of similar struggles and triumphs can offer comfort and perspective. These communities can be invaluable, providing a space to exchange advice, share burdens, and celebrate successes.

Through these connections, you gain insight into different parenting approaches, broadening your understanding. It also reinforces that there is no singular path to raising strong and courageous children. These interactions remind you that parenting is a shared experience. It is full of tests and trials, but know that you are part of a larger network sharing the same journey.

Self-Care

Parenting is demanding and requires constant emotional, physical, and mental energy. Without proper self-care, you risk burnout. Among other things this will diminish your patience, decision-making ability, and overall effectiveness in parenting.

Self-care should be a priority because it directly impacts your ability to care for your children optimally. By taking time to rest and recharge, you maintain your emotional stability and provide a loving environment for your children. This stability helps you model healthy coping mechanisms, teaching children by example the importance of balancing responsibilities with self-care. Children are highly perceptive. When they see you engaging in self-care, they learn to value their own needs and understand the importance of maintaining balance in life.

Self-care enables you to better meet the long-term demands of raising courageous, independent children. Neglecting personal needs over time can lead to chronic stress, health issues, and emotional exhaustion. This will compromise the quality of your parenting. By prioritizing your health and happiness, you are better equipped to overcome barriers and provide consistent support and guidance to your children. Self-care is not selfish; it is a vital investment in the entire family's well-being. It will ensure you can sustain your role as a loving, attentive caregiver for years to come.

Rest is a fundamental part of self-care and deserves special mention. Ensuring you get enough sleep is not a luxury, but a necessity. Rest and sleep allow your body and mind to repair, rejuvenate, and function at their best. Quality sleep improves cognitive performance, emotional regulation, and physical health. It will enable you to tackle daily challenges with clarity and resolve.

Beyond sleep, incorporating regular moments of relaxation throughout your day is also imperative. These pauses help recharge your mental and physical reserves. Prioritizing rest enhances your productivity and sets a calmer, more balanced tone for the day. It will reduce stress and foster a greater sense of overall peace and well-being.

Determining the best self-care strategies for you involves a combination of self-reflection and experimentation. But you must first understand your unique needs, preferences, and circumstances. Here's a step-by-step guide to help you get started with a self-care routine.

1. Assess Your Needs in Four Main Dimensions

Physical

Are you feeling fatigued, tense, or unwell?

How does your body feel throughout the day? Do you notice persistent tension or discomfort?

Are there specific times or activities that leave you feeling drained or energized?

Do you sleep well? If not, what might affect your sleep quality or quantity?

How do you feel after meals? Are there foods that leave you feeling sluggish or unwell?

Do you feel you have enough physical activity in your day? If not, what prevents you from moving more?

Are there any signals your body is giving (e.g., headaches, back pain, low energy) that you've been ignoring?

Emotional

Do you often feel stressed, overwhelmed, or emotionally drained?

Are there particular situations or people that consistently trigger stress or negative feelings?

How do you typically process your emotions—do you bottle them up, express them, or avoid them altogether?

When did you last feel joy or deep contentment, and what contributed to that experience?

Do you feel you have outlets for expressing your emotions, such as creative pursuits, conversations, or personal reflection?

What coping mechanisms do you rely on during stressful times? Are they effective?

Social

Are you feeling isolated or disconnected?

Do you feel connected to the people in your life, or do your relationships feel distant or unfulfilling?

When was the last time you felt truly supported or understood by someone else?

Do you avoid social interactions, and if so, why?

Are there people in your life who uplift you, and are you spending enough time with them?

Do you have time to meet new people or strengthen existing connections?

How do you feel after spending time with others—recharged, drained, or somewhere in between?

Spiritual

Do you feel a lack of purpose or connection?

Do you feel a sense of meaning or purpose in your life? If not, what might be missing?

When do you feel most at peace or deeply connected to something larger than yourself?

How often do you take time to reflect on your values, beliefs, or personal growth?

Are there practices or routines in your life that help you feel grounded and centered?

Do you feel in tune with nature, creativity, or other sources of inspiration and wonder?

Is there an aspect of your spiritual or inner life you've neglected or want to explore further?

2. **Reflect on what brings you joy and relaxation.** Think about activities that leave you feeling refreshed and fulfilled. This could be reading, painting, gardening, cooking, or even something as simple as taking a bath or listening to music.

3. **Consider your current lifestyle.** Your self-care practices need to fit within your daily life. If your schedule is tight, look for quick and accessible strategies, such as a five-minute mindfulness exercise or a brisk walk during lunch.

4. **Experiment with different strategies.** Try out various self-care activities to see what resonates with you. For example, test different exercise regimes (yoga, running, swimming) or relaxation techniques (deep breathing, progressive muscle relaxation). Pay attention to how you feel afterward. Does the activity leave you feeling calm, energized, or grounded?

5. **Listen to your body and mind.** Identify which areas need attention when you feel out of balance or depleted. If you're physically tired,

prioritize rest; if you're emotionally drained, focus on activities that bring joy or connection.

6. Set realistic goals. Start small and build consistent habits. Overloading yourself with too many strategies at once can be overwhelming and counterproductive.

7. Reevaluate periodically. Your needs and circumstances can change, so you must regularly reassess what works for you. What helped during a stressful period might not be as necessary during a calmer phase.

8. Seek feedback and inspiration. Talk to friends, family, or a therapist about their strategies. Hearing about others' practices can sometimes spark ideas you hadn't considered.

9. Trust your instincts. Self-care is deeply personal. If something feels good and aligns with your values and needs, it's likely a good fit for you—even if it doesn't work for others.

Summary

As you cultivate new self-care skills for yourself, you are modeling resilience for your children. You can pave the way for a nurturing and supportive family environment. The skills developed here ripple outwards, influencing your children's ability to navigate the world with vigor and adaptability.

By being intentional, open-minded, and self-aware, you can craft a self-care routine that protects your well-being and supports a more balanced life.

Keeping the Journey Going

Now that you have the tools to help your children thrive and grow into strong, confident adults, it's time to share what you've learned and help others discover the same guidance.

By leaving your honest opinion of *Raising Resilient Children* on Amazon, you're not just sharing your thoughts—you're lighting the way for other parents, caregivers, and teachers seeking to raise resilient kids.

Thank you for taking a moment to make a difference. Resilience isn't just something we teach—it's something we keep alive by sharing and supporting one another.

>>> Scan the QR code to leave your review on Amazon.

Your contribution matters more than you know. Thank you for being part of this mission!

With gratitude,

Lee Alexander

Conclusion

Raising resilient children is one of the greatest gifts you can give—not just to them, but to the world they will one day help shape. This is not about striving for perfection as a parent or expecting it from your children; it's about embracing the journey of growth, learning, and connection. Resilience is a complex web of skills, traits, and habits that can be taught, practiced, and perfected, in anyone, including you and your children.

It starts with a solid foundation of love, attachment to caregivers, safety, and stability. It includes emotional well-being, where understanding and expressing emotions leads to healthier relationships and self-awareness. It involves mindset, encouraging children to view difficulties as learning opportunities rather than obstacles to avoid.

Critical thinking and problem-solving play a role in being self-reliant and efficacious. Independence and autonomy in childhood set the stage for adult success. Creativity and adaptability are paramount in overcoming obstacles. Bouncing back from hardship determines who will continue to thrive well into adulthood and who will let life get the best of them.

As a parent, your character and emotional regulation significantly impact your children's development. Take time to understand your strengths and areas for improvement. Reflect on your attitudes and behaviors and how they shape your children's mindset. This ongoing self-reflection is vital for adapting parenting strategies to meet your children's evolving needs.

But the journey doesn't end here. It's a continuous process of learning and adapting. Now, it's time to implement these strategies. Create a personalized action plan for your family. Develop a resilience toolkit that includes the exercises and insights that resonate most with you and your children. This proactive approach will empower you to implement the ideas you've learned and tailor them to your unique family dynamic.

Nurturing resilience in your children is a gift you are giving them that sets the stage for lifelong success and emotional well-being. You are crafting a foundation of strength and adaptability that will serve your children throughout their lives. You are creating an environment where your children feel safe to explore, learn, and grow; they will be braver, stronger, and happier because of it. They'll carry these skills into their schooling, careers, and relationships, equipped to face life's inevitable challenges with certainty and courage.

Your dedication to this endeavor is a testament to your love for your children.

References

5Rights Foundation. (2024). *Digital Childhood*. Retrieved from https://5rightsfoundation.com/wp-content/uploads/2024/10/digital-childhood-final-report.pdf

Amato, P. R., & Fowler, F. (2002). Parenting practices, child adjustment, and family diversity. Journal of Marriage and Family, 64(3), 703–716. https://doi.org/10.1111/j.1741-3737.2002.00703.x

American Psychological Association. (1993). *The Origins of Attachment Theory: John Bowlby and Mary...* Retrieved from https://psycnet.apa.org/record/1993-01038-001

American Psychological Association. (2019). *Identifying Signs of Stress in Your Children and Teens*. Retrieved from https://www.apa.org/topics/stress/children

American Psychological Association. (2020, February 1). *Building Your Resilience*. Retrieved from https://www.apa.org/topics/resilience/building-your-resilience

American Psychological Association. (2024, March 21). *Nurturing Children Through Grief, With Help From Elmo and His Cousin, Jesse*. Retrieved from https://www.apa.org/topics/grief/nurturing-children-grief

American Psychological Association. (2024, October 22). *How to Help Children and Teens Manage Their Stress*. Retrieved from https://www.apa.org/topics/children/stress

American Psychological Association. (n.d.). *Resilience Guide for Parents and Teachers*. Retrieved from https://www.apa.org/topics/resilience/guide-parents-teachers

American Psychological Association. (n.d.). *Resilience*. Retrieved from https://dictionary.apa.org/resilience

American Psychological Association. (n.d.). *Self-Care*. Retrieved from https://www.apa.org/research-practice/self-care

American Society for Quality. (n.d.). *Five Whys and Five Hows*. Retrieved from https://asq.org/quality-resources/five-whys

Angoff, L. (n.d.). *Explaining Anxiety to Kids*. Explaining Brains. Retrieved from https://explainingbrains.com/explaining-anxiety/

Atkinson, W. W. (2013). *The Art of Logical Thinking*. Duke Classics.

Badegruber, B. (2006, August 21). *101 More Life Skills Games for Children: Learning, Growing, Getting Along (Ages 9-15)*. Hunter House.

BBC Bitesize. (n.d.). What is an algorithm? Retrieved January 19, 2025, from https://www.bbc.co.uk/bitesize/articles/z3whpv4

Be You. (n.d.). *Children's Risky Play and Mental Health Benefits.* Retrieved from https://beyou.edu.au/resources/news/risky-play-for-children-and-mental-health-benefits

Benjaidismas. (n.d.). 30 *Best Strategies of Fostering Independence in Children.* Conceive and Connect. Retrieved from https://conceiveandconnect.com/30-best-strategies-of-fostering-independence-in-children

Beyer, A. L. (2023, September 26). *An Age-By-Age Guide to Raising an Autonomous Kid: Be Less Controlling Now So They Can Be More Independent Later.* Lifehacker. Retrieved from https://lifehacker.com/an-age-by-age-guide-to-raising-an-autonomous-kid

Black Dog Institute. (n.d.). *How to Use Self-Care Planning to Improve Your Emotional Wellbeing, Even When You Don't Think You Need It.* Retrieved from https://www.blackdoginstitute.org.au/news/how-to-use-self-care-planning-to-improve-your-emotional-wellbeing

BMC Psychiatry. (2023). *Structural Model of Resilience Based on Parental Support.* Retrieved from https://bmcpsychiatry.biomedcentral.com/articles/10.1186/s12888-023-04678-z

Bonanno, G. A. (2004). *Loss, Trauma, and Human Resilience: Have We Underestimated the Human Capacity to Thrive After Extremely Aversive Events? American Psychologist, 59*(1), 20–28. https://doi.org/10.1037/0003-066X.59.1.20

Bransford, J. D., & Stein, B. S. (1984). *The IDEAL Problem-Solving Model.*

Bransford, J. D., & Stein, B. S. (1993). *The Ideal Problem Solver: A Guide for Improving Thinking, Learning, and Creativity* (2nd ed.). W. H. Freeman and Company. Retrieved from https://ouweb.tntech.edu/cat/pdf/useful_links/idealproblemsolver.pdf

Briggs, S. (2015, February 10). *25 Ways to Develop a Growth Mindset.* Open Colleges. Retrieved from https://www.opencolleges.edu.au/blogs/articles/25-ways-to-develop-a-growth-mindset-open-colleges

Brightwheel. (2023, April 7). *Autonomy in Child Development: Build Confident and Independent Children by Supporting Autonomy in Early Childhood.* Retrieved from https://brightwheel.com/blog/autonomy-in-child-development

Center on the Developing Child. (2019, January 22). *How to Motivate Children: Science-Based Approaches for Parents, Caregivers, and Teachers.* Harvard University. Retrieved from https://developingchild.harvard.edu/resources/how-to-motivate-children-science-based-approaches-for-parents-caregivers-and-teachers/

Chapman, G. (2012). *5 Love Languages*. Moody Publishing.

Chapman, G., & Campbell, R. (2016). The 5 Love Languages of Children. Chicago: Northfield Publishing.

Charity for Change. (n.d.). *Perseverance Is a Life-Long Skill Children Need*. Retrieved from https://charityforchange.org/perseverance-is-a-life-long-skill-children-need/

Cherry, K. (2024, July 14). *Cognitive Developmental Milestones: From Birth to Five Years*. Verywell Mind. Retrieved from https://www.verywellmind.com/cognitive-developmental-milestones-2795109

Cherry, K. (2024, July 3). *What Is Empathy? How It Helps Strengthen Our Relationships*. Verywell Mind. Retrieved from https://www.verywellmind.com/what-is-empathy-2795562

Child Mind Institute. (n.d.). *Helping Kids Make Decisions*. Retrieved from https://childmind.org/article/helping-kids-make-decisions/

Child Mind Institute. (n.d.). *How Can We Help Kids With Emotional Self-Regulation?* Retrieved from https://childmind.org/article/can-help-kids-self-regulation/

Child Mind Institute. (n.d.). *Talking to Kids About Bullying*. Retrieved from https://childmind.org

Cleveland Clinic. (2021, March 31). *Signs That Your Child May Need a Therapist*. Retrieved from https://health.clevelandclinic.org/signs-your-child-may-need-a-therapist/

Cleveland Clinic. (2023, August 3). *The Internet and Your Kids: 8 Tips for Keeping Safe Online*. Retrieved from https://health.clevelandclinic.org/internet-safety-for-kids

Cohen, S. S. (n.d.). *The Ultimate Internet Safety Guide for Kids*. Forbes. Retrieved from https://www.forbes.com/home-improvement/internet/child-internet-safety-guide/

Coloroso, B. (2003). *The Bully, the Bullied, and the Bystander*. Collins.

Common Sense Media. (2020, June 4). *What Is Digital Literacy?* Retrieved from https://www.commonsensemedia.org/articles/what-is-digital-literacy

Confident Parents Confident Kids. (2021, July 1). *Understanding the Social and Emotional Development of Tween-Agers*. Retrieved from https://confidentparentsconfidentkids.org/2021/07/01/understanding-the-social-and-emotional-development-of-tween-agers/

Cook Center for Human Connection. (n.d.). *9 Ways to Teach Children How to Handle Peer Pressure*. Retrieved from https://cookcenter.org/9-ways-to-teach-children-how-to-handle-peer-pressure/

Coursera Staff. (2024, November 21). *What Is Active Listening and How Can You Improve This Key Skill?* Coursera. Retrieved from https://www.coursera.org/articles/active-listening

Culbertson, S. (n.d.). *Teaching Youth Real-World Problem-Solving Skills.* Retrieved from https://www.linkedin.com/pulse/teaching-youth-real-world-problem-solving-skills-steven-culbertson

Cyberbullying Research Center. (n.d.). *Preventing Cyberbullying.* Retrieved from https://cyberbullying.org

Developing Minds. (2020, October 21). *12 Practical Steps to Support Children and Young People Who Have Experienced Grief and Loss.* Retrieved from https://developingminds.net.au/blog/2020/10/21/2-practical-steps-to-support-children-and-young-people-who-have-experienced-grief-and-loss

Doinita, N. E., & Mariab, N. D. (2015). *Attachment and Parenting Styles.* Procedia - Social and Behavioral Sciences, 203, 199–204.

Duckworth, A. L. (2016). *Grit: The Power of Passion and Perseverance.* Scribner.

Dweck, C. S. (2006). *Mindset: The New Psychology of Success.* Random House.

Edutopia. (n.d.). *Boosting Resilience Through Creativity.* Retrieved from https://www.edutopia.org/article/boosting-resilience-through-creativity/

Ehmke, R. (n.d.). *Helping Children Deal With Grief.* Child Mind Institute. Retrieved from https://childmind.org/article/helping-children-deal-grief/

EI Excellence. (2015, June 3). *Using Reflective Questions to Empower Parents: A Table Talk Wednesday Recap.* Retrieved from https://www.eiexcellence.org/using-reflective-questions-to-empower-parents-a-table-talk-wednesday-recap/

Elias, M. J. (2022, November 2). *Social and Emotional Skill Progression in Preschool.* Edutopia. Retrieved from https://www.edutopia.org/article/social-and-emotional-skill-progression-in-preschool

ERIC. (2020). *Promoting Social and Emotional Competencies in Early Childhood.* Retrieved from https://files.eric.ed.gov/fulltext/EJ1240550.pdf

Evans, J. (2024, December 2). *175 of the Best Self-Reflection Questions to Ask Yourself.* Healthy Happy Impactful. Retrieved from https://healthyhappyimpactful.com/self-reflection-questions/

Fleming, N. D. (1987). *The VARK Model of Learning Styles.*

Framework Garage. (n.d.). *From Toyota to Analytics: The Evolution of the 5 Whys Framework.* Retrieved from https://www.frameworkgarage.com/post/from-toyota-to-analytics-the-evolution-of-the-5-whys-framework

French American Academy. (n.d.). *6 Tips for Fostering Independence and Autonomy in Children.* Retrieved from https://faacademy.org/6-tips-for-fostering-independence-and-autonomy-in-children/

Gardner, H. (1983). *Frames of Mind: The Theory of Multiple Intelligences.* Basic Books.

Garey, J. (2024, March 8). *Teaching Kids How to Deal With Conflict: Tips for Building Lifelong Skills.* Child Mind Institute. Retrieved from https://childmind.org/article/teaching-kids-how-to-deal-with-conflict/

Garraway, R. (2023, June 13). *Effective Communication and Empathy: How to Communicate Better With Social Skills and Confidence to Create Lasting Relationships and Connect Effortlessly.* Independently Published.

GRIP Learning. (2024, November 15). *7 Ways to Help Your Child Learn From Failure.* Retrieved from https://grip-learning.com/blog/7-ways-to-help-your-child-learn-from-failure/

Grover, S. (2016, April 10). *7 Positive Ways to Help Kids Manage Disappointment.* Psychology Today. Retrieved from https://www.psychologytoday.com/us/blog/when-kids-call-the-shots/201604/7-positive-ways-to-help-kids-manage-disappointment

Grumet, J. (2019). *Modern Attachment Parenting.*

Harvard Center on the Developing Child. (n.d.). *How to Motivate Children: Science-Based Approaches for Parents, Caregivers, and Teachers.* Retrieved from https://developingchild.harvard.edu/resources/how-to-motivate-children-science-based-approaches-for-parents-caregivers-and-teachers/

Healing Collective Therapy. (n.d.). *10 Family Therapy Activities for Building Relationships.* Retrieved from https://healingcollectivetherapy.com/resources/family-therapy-activities

Heart-Mind Online. (n.d.). *How to Model Regulation as a Parent or Caregiver.* Retrieved from https://heartmindonline.org/resources/regulation-is-connection-how-to-model-regulation-as-a-parent-or-caregiver

Henley, D. (2018). *Creativity: Why It Matters.* Elliott & Thompson.

Holland, K. (2018, July 30). *Are You an Extrovert? Here's How to Tell.* Healthline. Retrieved from https://www.healthline.com/health/what-is-an-extrovert

Holland, K., & Raypole, C. (2021, November 9). *What an Introvert Is — and Isn't.* Healthline. Retrieved from https://www.healthline.com/health/what-is-an-introvert

Hunter, S. (2021). *Emotional Intelligence Mastery: Develop Self-Discipline, Overcome Procrastination, and Overthinking.* Syed Publishing Co.

InsideOut Mastery. (2024, January 16). *420 Self-Reflection Questions for Personal Growth: Unlock a New You.* Retrieved from https://insideoutmastery.com/self-reflection-questions/

IRB Media. (2022). *Summary of Richard Louv's Last Child in the Woods.* IRB Media.

Kaizen4U. (2023). *The 5 Whys.* Retrieved from https://www.kaizen4u.com/post/5-whys

Kataria, P. (2022, January). *Resilience and Gender Differences. Clinical Psychology,* 10(Jan/Feb). Amity University, Noida, India.

Katz, R., & Hadani, H. S. (2022). *The Emotionally Intelligent Child: Effective Strategies for Parenting Self-Aware, Cooperative, and Well-Balanced Kids.* New Harbinger Publications.

Kharbach, M. (2024, September 7). 80 *Learning Reflection Questions for Students.* Educators Technology. Retrieved from https://www.educatorstechnology.com/2023/06/80-learning-reflection-questions-for-students.html

Laff, R., & Ruiz, W. (2019). *Child, Family, and Community.* College of the Canyons. Retrieved from https://drive.google.com/file/d/1B4Y2EEp7HoECRBh_vXP3BCrg84QYOnjD/view

Lahoti, I. A. (2023, May 15). *Parents' Attitudes and Beliefs: Their Impact on Children's Development.* Parenting. Retrieved from https://blog.growthbest.com/parents-attitudes-and-beliefs-their-impact-on-childrens-development/

Lasting Leaps Limited. (2015). *A Jooser Guide to Daniel Goleman Emotional Intelligence: Why It Can Matter More Than IQ.*

Life Skills Advocate. (n.d.). 7 *Cognitive Flexibility Strategies to Support Your Adolescent.* Retrieved from https://lifeskillsadvocate.com/blog/7-flexible-thinking-strategies-to-support-your-teen-or-young-adult/

LoBue, V. (2022, March 7). *How Parental Stress Can Affect a Child's Health.* Psychology Today. Retrieved from https://www.psychologytoday.com/us/blog/the-baby-scientist/202203/how-parental-stress-can-affect-childs-health

Lomax, F. (2020). *Your Creative Child: A Parent's Guide.* Frank Lomax.

Marie, S. (2022, June 23). *The Importance of Validating Your Child's Feelings.* PsychCentral. Retrieved from https://psychcentral.com/blog/the-powerful-parenting-tool-of-validation

Marrow, S., & Powell, M. M. (n.d.). *Communication, Resilience, and the Family.* Retrieved from https://artshumanitieshawaii.org/assets/marrow%2C--sherilyn-ph.d-and-mary-m.-powell---m.a-communication%2C-resilience-and-the-family.pdf

Marter, J. (2023, March 5). *A Tool to Assess and Improve Your Self-Care Practices.* Psychology Today. Retrieved from https://www.psychologytoday.com/intl/blog/mental-wealth/202302/a-tool-to-assess-and-improve-your-self-care-practices

Martinelli, K. (n.d.). *How Can We Help Kids With Transitions?* Child Mind Institute. Retrieved from https://childmind.org/article/how-can-we-help-kids-with-transitions/

Mindset Works. (n.d.). *The Growth Mindset: What Is Growth Mindset?* Retrieved from https://www.mindsetworks.com/science/

Morin, A. (n.d.). *Social and Emotional Skills at Different Ages.* Understood.org. Retrieved from https://www.understood.org/en/articles/social-and-emotional-skills-what-to-expect-at-different-ages

NAEYC. (n.d.). *Supporting Children's Reflection With Phones and Tablets.* Retrieved from https://www.naeyc.org/resources/pubs/tyc/jun2015/supporting-childrens-reflection

National Bullying Prevention Center (PACER). (n.d.). *Build Self-Esteem and Resilience.* Retrieved from https://www.pacer.org/bullying

National Center for Biotechnology Information. (n.d.). *Introduction to Children's Attachment.* Retrieved from https://www.ncbi.nlm.nih.gov/books/NBK356196/

National Education Association. (n.d.). *Prevent Bullying in Schools.* Retrieved from https://www.nea.org

National Scientific Council on the Developing Child (2012). The Science of Neglect: The Persistent Absence of Responsive Care Disrupts the Developing Brain: Working Paper No. 12. Retrieved from http://www.developingchild.harvard.edu.

NeuroLaunch Editorial Team. (2024, October 18). *Healthy Emotional Expression: Cultivating Emotional Intelligence for Well-Being.* Retrieved from https://neurolaunch.com/healthy-emotional-expression/

NeuroLaunch Editorial Team. (2024, September 22). *Parental Influence on Child Behavior: Shaping Future Generations. Developmental Psychology and Behavior.* Retrieved from https://neurolaunch.com/how-do-parents-influence-their-childs-behavior/

NeuroLaunch Editorial Team. (2024, September 30). *Emotional Intelligence History: From Concept to Global Phenomenon.* Retrieved from https://neurolaunch.com/history-of-emotional-intelligence/

Nhan, H. (n.d.). *How Do Parenting Styles, Parental Gender, and Culture Impact Children's Mental Health and Behavior? The Scholarly Journal of North Hennepin Community College.* Retrieved from https://northernlight.nhcc.edu/northlight/parenting-styles-behavior

NPR. (2022, March 14). *Time Management Tips for Busy Working Parents: Life Kit.* Retrieved from https://www.npr.org/2022/03/14/1086480869/parents-are-exhausted-these-strategies-can-help-you-build-support-and-win-back-t

Parenting Science. (n.d.). *Teaching Critical Thinking: An Evidence-Based Guide.* Retrieved from https://parentingscience.com/teaching-critical-thinking/

PBS. (n.d.). *How to Help Kids Cope With Disappointment.* Retrieved from https://www.pbs.org/parents/thrive/how-to-help-kids-cope-with-disappointment

Penn State Extension. (2023, December 4). *Learning Through Failure: How You Can Help Your Child.* Retrieved from https://extension.psu.edu/learning-through-failure-how-you-can-help-your-child/

Positive Action Team. (2024, October 7). *Empowering Students With Effective Decision-Making Skills: A How-to Guide.* Retrieved from https://www.positiveaction.net/blog/empowering-students-with-effective-decision-making-skills

Price-Mitchell, M. (n.d.). *Teaching for Life Success: Why Resourcefulness Matters.* Retrieved from https://www.edutopia.org/blog/8-pathways-why-resourcefulness-matters-marilyn-price-mitchell

PsychCentral. (n.d.). *The Difference Between Mourning and Grieving.* Retrieved from https://psychcentral.com/health/mourning-vs-grief

PubMed Central. (2009). *Peer Influence in Children and Adolescents: Crossing the Line.* Retrieved from https://www.ncbi.nlm.nih.gov/pmc/articles/PMC2747364/

PubMed Central. (2016). *Parenting Stress and Child Behavior Problems.* Retrieved from https://pmc.ncbi.nlm.nih.gov/articles/PMC4861150/

PubMed Central. (2017). *Cyberbullying in Children and Youth: Implications for Mental Health.* Retrieved from https://pmc.ncbi.nlm.nih.gov/articles/PMC5455867/

PubMed Central. (2021). *Curiosity in Childhood and Adolescence—What Can We Learn?* Retrieved from https://pmc.ncbi.nlm.nih.gov/articles/PMC8363506/

PubMed Central. (2022). *Relevance for Mental Health Among School-Age Youths.* Retrieved from https://pmc.ncbi.nlm.nih.gov/articles/PMC9083540/

PubMed Central. (2023). *Cognitive Behavioral Stress Management for Parents.* Retrieved from https://www.ncbi.nlm.nih.gov/pmc/articles/PMC9999161/

QuizGecko. (n.d.). *Parenting Styles and Child Development Quiz.* Retrieved from https://quizgecko.com/learn/parenting-styles-and-child-development-quiz-xah5w7

ReadyKids Team. (n.d.). *Problem Solving for Kids: How-To Guide, Activities & Strategies.* Retrieved from https://readykids.com.au/kids-problem-solving/

Reboot Foundation. (n.d.). *The Parents' Guide to Critical Thinking.* Retrieved from https://reboot-foundation.org/resource/parent-guide/

Reference Staff. (2015, August 4). *What Is a Reflective Question?* Reference.com. Retrieved from https://www.reference.com/world-view/reflective-question-3e40707fadd3eecd

Riggs, J. (n.d.). *Play to Learn: Harnessing the Power of Gamification for Maximum Learning Potential.* Digital Alchemy.

Romani, P. (2024, May 15). *Helping Kids Bounce Back From Failure: Practical Strategies for Teaching Resilience*. Peartree School. Retrieved from https://peartree.school/teaching-resilience-to-children-tips/

Rosenberg, M. B. (2003). *Nonviolent Communication: A Language of Life*. PuddleDancer Press.

Rozon, D. (2023, October 17). *Teaching Emotional Regulation to Children: A Guide for Parents*. Elements Psychology. Retrieved from https://elementspsychology.ca/teaching-emotional-regulation-to-children-a-guide-for-parents/

Sahlberg, P., & Doyle, W. (2019). *Let the Children Play: How More Play Will Save Our Schools and Help Children Thrive*. Oxford University Press.

Sahni, A. (2024, August 17). *History of Emotional Intelligence: Origins, Evolution, and Background*. Kapable. Retrieved from https://kapable.club/blog/emotional-intelligence/history-of-emotional-intelligence/

Schaffner, A. K. (2020, September 16). *Perseverance in Psychology: Meaning, Importance & Books*. Positive Psychology. Retrieved from https://positivepsychology.com/perseverance/

Seabury, T. (n.d.). *Sakichi Toyoda and the 5 Whys*. Retrieved from https://www.seauryperformance.com/post/toyoda-and-the-5-whys

Severson Sisters. (2015, August 21). *Supergirl Guide to Peer Pressure: An Action Plan to Create Your Own Safe and Fabulous Place in the World*. Morgan James Publishing.

SickKids Staff. (n.d.). *Social and Emotional Development in School-Age Children*. AboutKidsHealth. Retrieved from https://www.aboutkidshealth.ca/social-and-emotional-development-in-school-age-children

Snyder, R. (2019). *Decisive Intuition*. Red Wheel Weiser.

Springer. (n.d.). *Enhancing Resiliency in Girls and Boys: A Case for Gender-Specific Adolescent Prevention Programming*. Retrieved from https://link.springer.com/article/10.1007/BF02407231

Status.net. (n.d.). *Adaptability: 25 Performance Review Phrases Examples*. Retrieved from https://status.net/articles/adaptability-performance-review-phrases-paragraphs-examples/

StopBullying.gov. (n.d.). *Respond to Bullying*. Retrieved from https://www.stopbullying.gov

Storm, A. (2023, March 14). *The 7 Main Types of Learning Styles (and How to Teach to Them)*. Thinkific. Retrieved from https://www.thinkific.com/blog/learning-styles

Sun, J., & Stewart, D. (2007). *Age and Gender Effects on Resilience in Children and Adolescents*. International Journal of Mental Health Promotion. © The Clifford Beers Foundation.

Sutton, J. (2016, October 4). *Martin Seligman's Positive Psychology Theory*. Positive Psychology. Retrieved from https://positivepsychology.com/positive-psychology-theory/

Sutton, J. (2019, January 3). *What Is Resilience, and Why Is It Important to Bounce Back?* Positive Psychology. Retrieved from https://positivepsychology.com/what-is-resilience/

Taibbi, R. (2024, April 18). *The Art of Compromise.* Psychology Today. Retrieved from https://www.psychologytoday.com/us/blog/fixing-families/202404/the-art-of-compromise

Tava Health. (2024, June 25). *The Essential Guide to Self-Care: Strategies, Benefits, and When to Seek Help.* Retrieved from https://www.tavahealth.com/resources/self-care-tips-strategies

The Decision Lab. (n.d.). Confirmation bias. Retrieved January 19, 2025, from https://thedecisionlab.com/biases/confirmation-bias

The Family Centre. (2024, April 1). *How to Teach Problem-Solving Skills to Your Child: A Guide for Every Age.* Retrieved from https://www.familycentre.org/news/post/how-to-teach-problem-solving-skills-to-your-child-a-guide-for-every-age

The Therapist Parent. (n.d.). *Helping Children Grow Through Setbacks.* Retrieved from https://www.thetherapistparent.com/post/helping-children-grow-through-set-backs

TheVibeVenture. (2023). *Fostering Independence in Children: A Comprehensive Guide to Empowerment.* Retrieved from https://www.bulbapp.io/p/3e34e71c-4048-4f78-9a5a-a0d7f9a89938

ThinkPsych. (2023, March 9). *Expanding Emotional Vocabulary for Children.* Retrieved from https://thinkpsych.com/blogs/posts/emotional-vocabulary-for-children

Tough, P. (2012). *How Children Succeed.* HarperCollins.

Turner, S., Norman, E., & Zunz, S. (1995). *Enhancing Resiliency in Girls and Boys: A Case for Gender-Specific Adolescent Prevention Programming. Journal of Primary Prevention, 16,* 25–38. https://doi.org/10.1007/BF02407231

U.S. News & World Report. (n.d.). *How to Build Digital Literacy for Your K-8 Child.* Retrieved from https://www.usnews.com/education/k12/articles/how-to-build-digital-literacy-for-your-k-8-child

UNICEF. (n.d.). *How to Discipline Your Child the Smart and Healthy Way.* Retrieved from https://www.unicef.org/parenting/child-care/how-discipline-your-child-smart-and-healthy-way

University of Kansas Health System. (n.d.). *Why Is Emotional Expression Important?* Retrieved from https://www.kansashealthsystem.com/health-resources/turning-point/programs/resilience-toolbox/emotional-expression/why-is-emotional-expression-important

Uplift Kids. (n.d.). *Growth Mindset: Cultivating a Sense of Abundance.* Retrieved from https://upliftkids.org/growth-mindset/

Vallejo, M. (2024). *A Guide to Conflict Resolution for Kids*. Mental Health Center Kids. Retrieved from https://mentalhealthcenterkids.com/blogs/articles/conflict-resolution-for-kids/

Vanegas, Y. (2024, November 26). *3 Ways to Help Children Deal With Peer Pressure*. Psychology Today. Retrieved from https://www.psychologytoday.com/ca/blog/its-not-just-about-the-food/202411/3-ways-to-help-children-deal-with-peer-pressure

Vermani, M. (2022, July 9). *Resilience: What It Is and Why We Need It When the Going Gets Tough*. Psychology Today. Retrieved from https://www.psychologytoday.com/us/blog/deeper-wellness/202207/resilience-what-it-is-and-why-we-need-it

Very Special Tales. (2024, May 2). *50 Best Stress-Relief Games and Activities for Students*. Retrieved from https://veryspecialtales.com/stress-relief-games-and-activities-for-students/

Watson Institute. (2025). *Social Skills to Handle Peer Pressure*. Retrieved from https://www.thewatsoninstitute.org/resource/i-can-handle-peer-pressure/

We Are Teachers. (n.d.). *25 Growth Mindset Activities to Inspire Confidence in Kids*. Retrieved from https://www.weareteachers.com/growth-mindset/

WebMD. (n.d.). *Age-Appropriate Chores for Children*. Retrieved from https://www.webmd.com/parenting/features/chores-for-children

Weir, K. (2017, September). *Maximizing Children's Resilience*. Monitor on Psychology, 48(8). Retrieved from https://www.apa.org/monitor/2017/09/cover-resilience

WFMCH Health. (2024, September 17). *Navigating Peer Pressure: How to Help Your Kids Make Positive Choices*. Pediatric Health Care. Retrieved from https://wfmchealth.org/pediatric-health-care/navigating-peer-pressure-how-to-help-your-kids-make-positive-choices/

Whole Child Counseling. (n.d.). *How to Teach Self-Awareness Skills to Children*. Retrieved from https://www.wholechildcounseling.com/post/how-to-teach-self-awareness-skills-to-children

WholeHearted School Counseling. (2023). *12 Essential Conflict Resolution Skills for Kids: Helping Children Become Independent Problem-Solvers*. Retrieved from https://wholeheartedschoolcounseling.com/2023/05/05/12-conflict-resolution-skills-for-kids-helping-children-become-independent-problem-solvers/

Wilson, C. R. (2022). *14 Conflict Resolution Strategies for the Workplace*. Positive Psychology. Retrieved from https://positivepsychology.com/conflict-resolution-in-the-workplace/

Also by Lee Alexander

Comprehensive Guide to Co-parenting With a Narcissist: Solutions to Protect Your Children, Maintain Boundaries, Prepare for Legal and Financial Battles, and Start Rebuilding

Comprehensive Guide to Co-parenting With a Narcissist: Companion Workbook

Printed in Dunstable, United Kingdom